Maximum Calves

a manual of synergistic weight training for the calf muscles

from Health For Life

Also by ***Health For Life:***

- **Legendary Abs**
- **Beyond Legendary Abs**
  A synergistic performance guide to Legendary Abs and SynerAbs
- **Power ForeArms!**
- **The Human Fuel Handbook**
  Nutrition for Peak Athletic Performance
- **SynerAbs:** 6 Minutes to a Flatter Stomach
- **SynerShape:** A Scientific Weight Loss Guide
- **SynerStretch:** For Whole Body Flexibility
- **The Psychology of Weight Loss:**
  A Guided Introspection
- **Secrets of Advanced Bodybuilders**
  A manual of synergistic weight training for the whole body
- **Secrets of Advanced Bodybuilders, Supplement #1**

Please Note:

This program contains exercises that, depending on your physical condition, may be hazardous to your health. Consult with your doctor before attempting these exercises.

User assumes all risk for performing the exercises described in this course. **Use of this course constitutes a covenant not to bring any lawsuit or action for injury caused by performing exercises illustrated in this course.**

ISBN 0-944831-16-8

Health For Life
8033 Sunset Blvd., Suite 483
Los Angeles, CA 90046
(213) 450-0070

Thank you for ordering Health For Life's *Maximum Calves!*

Maximum Calves is a powerful tool for a broad spectrum of athletes. It features two complete programs: The first delivers MASS; the second, unshakable stability and lightning-fast footwork. And neither involves endless sets of Standing Calf Raises.

Over two years in the making, **Maximum Calves** integrates the latest research in biomechanics with the practical experiences of serious bodybuilders, martial artists, and other athletes.

The program's efficiency is the result of optimization at every level: exercise selection, performance, sequence, and timing. Indeed, the *details* of performance and the *specific way the exercises are combined* are every bit as important as the exercises themselves.

How can that be?

Certain exercises work together to produce results greater than just the sum of the results of the individual exercises. This is *Synergism,* the basis for all Health For Life courses. Using the synergism principle, **Maximum Calves** can dramatically increase gains while reducing calf workout time to just fifteen minutes, twice a week. And it only takes *that* long at the program's highest level!

Maximum Calves begins with a thorough explanation of the biomechanical principles involved. Then come illustrated descriptions of the exercises. Next are the routines themselves, each featuring a progression of levels so you can start at the proper intensity for your level of experience. You'll also find a complete calf flexibility program included to keep you from tightening up as you increase strength and/or mass. Finally, to ensure you get the most out of the routines, the course covers the specifics of schedule: how much, how often.

Good luck...and get ready for a calf burn you won't believe!

☆ ☆ ☆

CALF MUSCLES AND THEIR ASSOCIATED MOVEMENTS

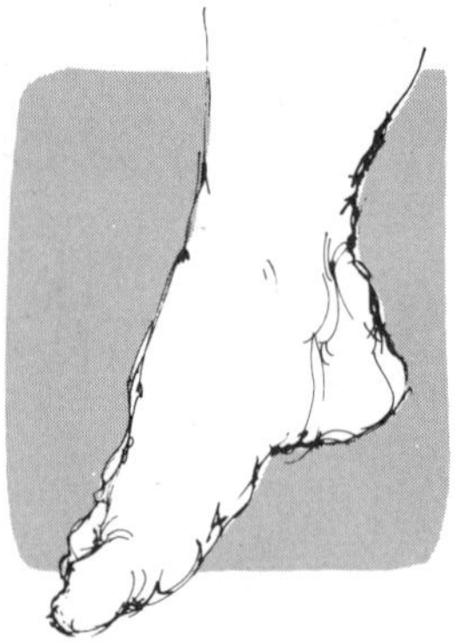

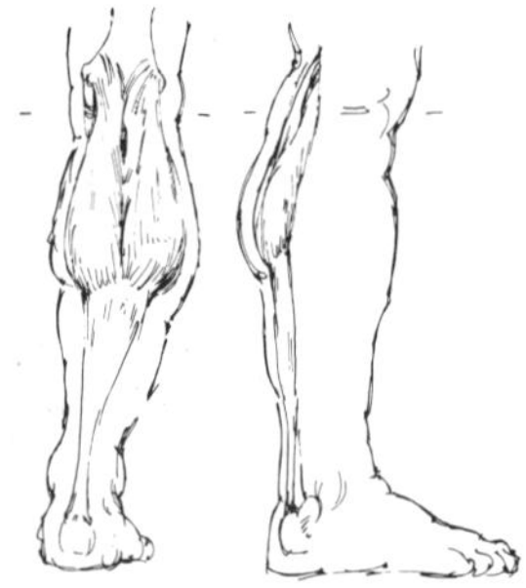

a. Plantar Flexion
involves...

Gastrocnemius

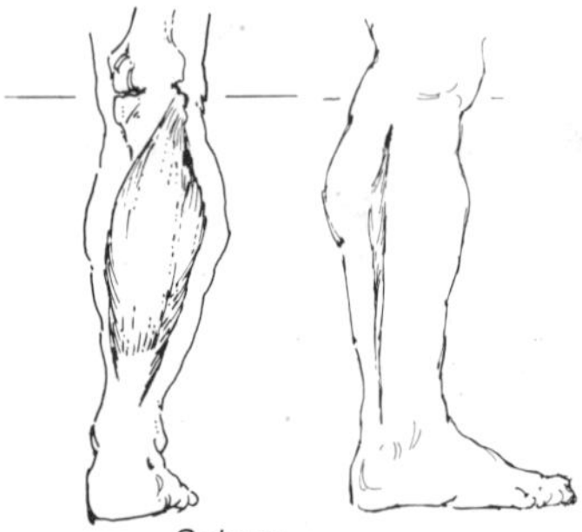

Soleus

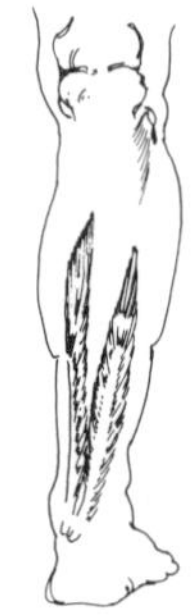

Flexor Hallucis & Flexor Digitorum

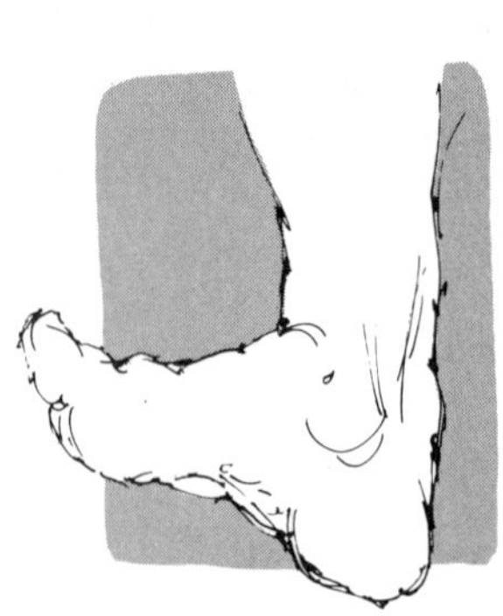

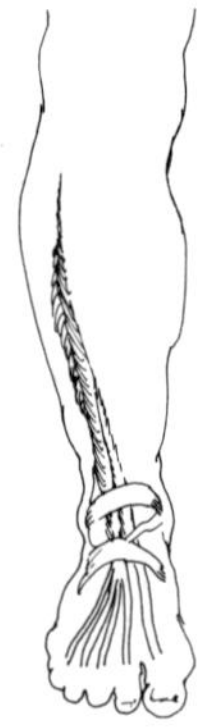

b. Dorsiflexion
involves...

Extensor Hallucis & Extensor Digitorum

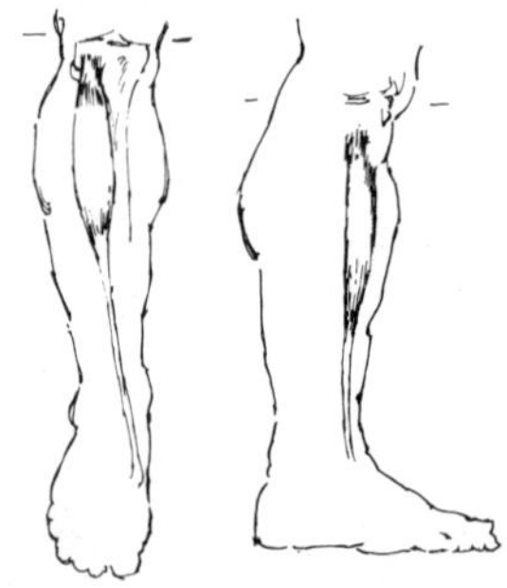

Anterior Tibialis

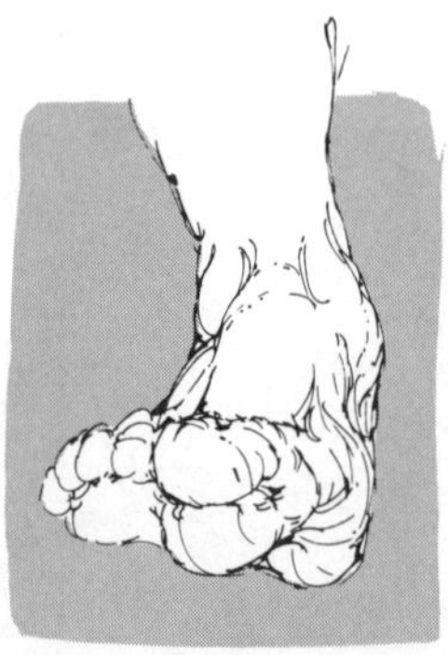

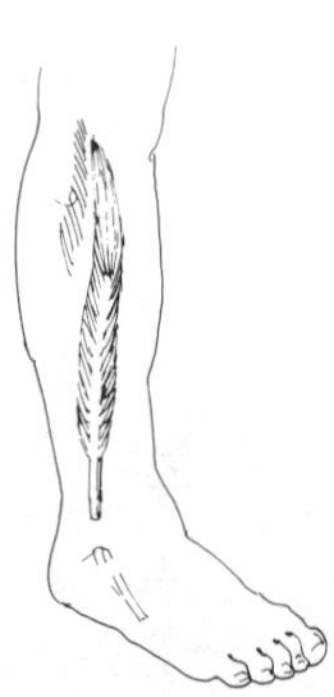

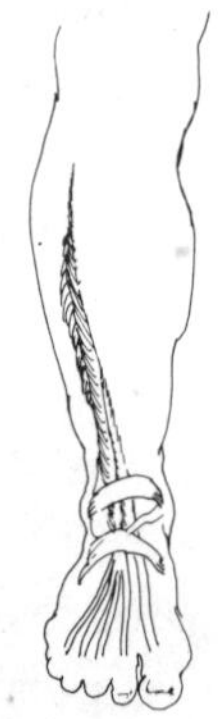

c. Pronation
involves...

Peroneus

Extensor Hallucis & Extensor Digitorum

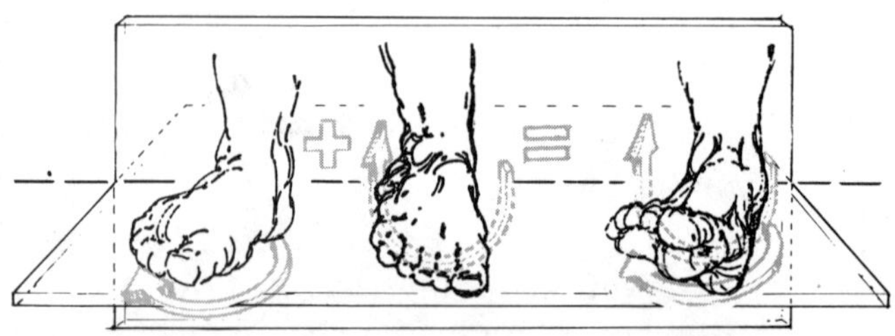

Abduction **Eversion** **Pronation**

Pronation *is actually a movement in two planes. It is a combination of two other movements:* ***Abduction*** *(turning the foot out) and* ***Eversion*** *(rolling the foot out).*

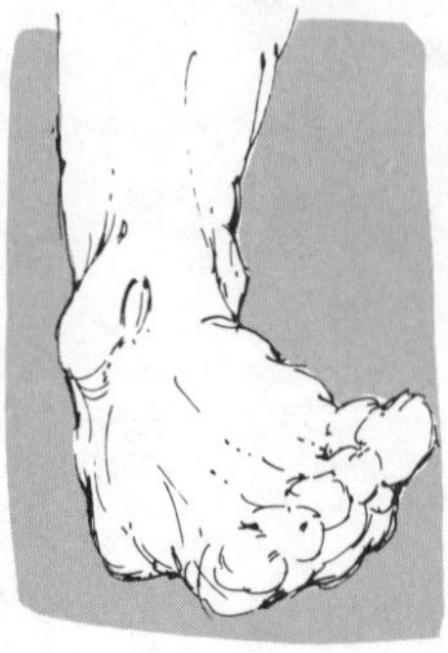

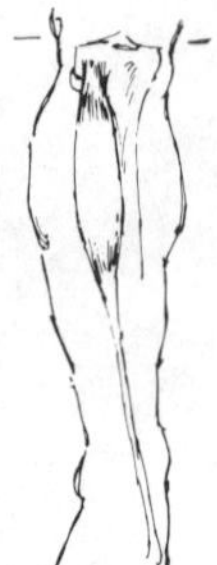

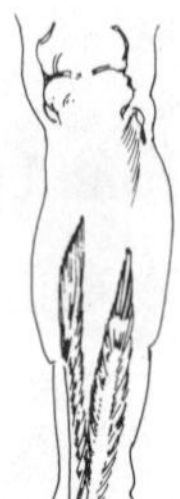

d. Supination
involves...

Anterior Tibialis

Flexor Hallucis & Flexor Digitorum

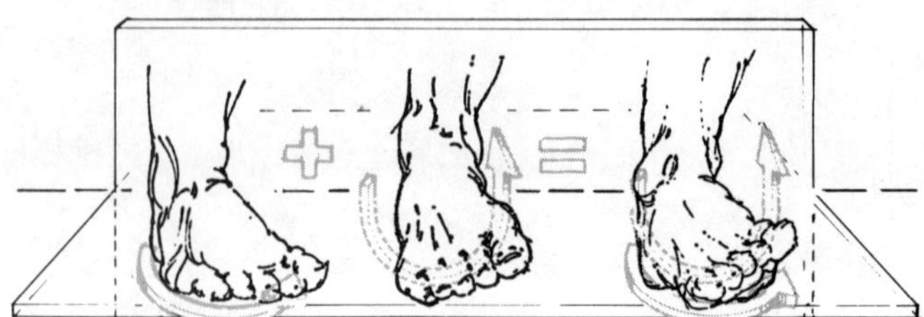

Adduction **Inversion** **Supination**

Supination *is also a movement in two planes. It is a combination of two other movements:* ***Adduction*** *(turning the foot in) and* ***Inversion*** *(rolling the foot in).*

IRENE DICONTI-MCKINNISS

THE THEORY

WHAT DOES WHAT

If you're an athlete whose success depends on fast footwork, strong thighs and great technique can do little to compensate for the instability resulting from weak calves. And if you're a bodybuilder—well, consider how many contests are lost by competitors whose only deficiency is below the knees!

In developing strong and/or massive calves, you should work for *balanced strength* around your ankle joints. Before we can talk about that, though, we must briefly touch on movements generated by the calf muscles.

The Moves

The calf muscles are responsible for all movements of the ankle and toes. For training purposes, we need only be concerned with ankle movements.

There are basically four, grouped in pairs:

plantar flexion / dorsiflexion

— and —

pronation / supination.

Plantar flexion is more commonly referred to as *pointing your toes*—which is a little strange since it's not a movement of the toes at all. It involves flexing your ankle so the front of your foot moves down, away from your shin (Fig. 1-a).

Dorsiflexion is the opposite of plantar flexion. It involves flexing your ankle so the front of your foot moves up, toward your shin (Fig. 1-b).

Pronation involves rolling your ankle so your toes move away from your body's centerline (Fig. 1-c).

And finally, **supination** is the opposite of pronation: rolling your ankle so your toes move in toward the centerline (Fig. 1-d).

If you want to get picky, *pronation* and *supination* can each be broken down into two component movements, and for the sticklers for biomechanical detail we have done so in the box on the opposite page. However, since the foot rarely—if ever—just executes any one of those component movements, this distinction is not that useful outside the biomechanics classroom.

We'll stick to the basic ankle movements listed above.

The Muscles

Each of these four main ankle movements is the result of several calf muscles working together in **muscle groups.** For the most part, it will satisfy our needs to refer to these groups in terms of their functions. For example, we'll call the calf muscles that plantar flex the ankle the *plantar flexors*, those that dorsiflex the ankle the *dorsiflexors*, and so on.

We will need to make specific reference to three individual calf muscles: *soleus, gastrocnemius*, and *anterior tibialis*.

The first two—soleus and gastroc—are the main plantar flexors. In Figure 1-a, notice that although both muscles lie in the upper rear portion of the calf, *only the gastroc crosses the knee joint*. This fact is going to be significant later on.

The third is the anterior tibialis, which runs up the front of the calf next to the shin bone (Fig. 1-b). It's often ignored by bodybuilders, but shouldn't be. Well-developed anterior tibialis muscles can make the difference between merely good legs and legs that look as if they should be part of a Greek statue!

Any comprehensive calf program should aim to develop all the major calf muscles. Achieving **balanced development** requires devoting **equal effort** to the opposing muscle groups at the ankle (i.e. plantar flexors and dorsiflexors, pronators and supinators). These paired groups work against one another to provide stability much like guy-wires on opposite sides of a tent pole.

Only such a balanced approach will generate **functional strength**—and ripped, massive calves as well.

As additional benefits, balanced calf development will:

- increase footwork speed and overall stability—ingredients essential to the success of many different kinds of athletic endeavors
- reduce the risk of spraining your ankles during athletic performance.

- **The calves are responsible for two pairs of opposing ankle movements:**
  - ❑ **plantar flexion / dorsiflexion**
  - ❑ **pronation / supination**
- **Each movement is the result of several calf muscles working together in *muscle groups***
- **Balanced development of the opposing muscle groups dramatically increases functional strength, footwork speed, and ankle stability. It also decreases risk of ankle injury.**

THE FATIGUE/TENSION PRINCIPLE

Exercise physiologists have spent a lot of time trying to figure out what makes muscles grow. They've understood pieces of the puzzle for some time—the idea of **progressive resistance**, for example. We all know constantly forcing ourselves to lift more than we think we can is essential for growth.

We also know **pace** is important. All three of the following limit growth: doing individual reps too slowly within a set; resting too long between sets; resting too long between workouts.

These two principles—progressive resistance and pace—have produced the well-known formula for muscle growth/strength increase:

- use a weight with which you can only do six to eight reps
- do three to five sets
- work moderately fast
- train a bodypart no more than three times per week.

But is that all there is to it?

No!

Research shows that resistance, number of reps per set, and pace are not independent of one another. It's not a question of just determining the **optimal resistance**, **number of reps**, or **best pace**. These three are inextricably intertwined. For a particular amount of resistance and number of reps, there is a maximum allowable rest length that will still foster growth. For a particular rest length, there is a minimum amount of resistance and number of reps necessary to foster growth.

If, for example, you do six to eight reps using 80% of your max weight, you must rest no more than 30 seconds between sets to sustain maximum growth. If, on the other hand, you use 95% of your max, you can rest about one minute and still sustain maximum growth.*

Resistance, number of reps, and pace act together.

Resistance creates a particular **tension level** in a muscle. The greater the weight you lift, the greater the tension level:

Greater resistance (more weight) ⟶ Higher *tension* level

The number of reps you perform, speed with which you perform them, and the time between sets act together to create a particular **fatigue level**. The faster you work, and the less time between sets, the higher the level of fatigue.

Greater rep speed, shorter rests between sets ⟶ Higher *fatigue* level

In combination, these two factors determine your **Fatigue/Tension Level**. This new term is a way of expressing that it is the combined effect of fatigue and tension that reflects how "hard" you have worked. We can say...

***Fatigue* in conjunction with *tension* ⟶ Fatigue/Tension Level**

Increase your pace (faster reps, less time between sets), and it takes less tension (less weight) to achieve the same Fatigue/Tension level. Decrease your pace (slower reps, more

* Numbers listed are for the intermediate bodybuilder—one to two years' training. These numbers change depending on, among other things, the lifter's experience.

time between sets) and it takes more tension (more weight) to achieve the same Fatigue/Tension level.

Now for the interesting part. It turns out muscle growth depends not only on fatigue, not only on tension, but on **surpassing a particular Fatigue/Tension level** we'll call the **Fatigue/Tension *Threshold*. Unless your exercise scheme (resistance, number of reps, and pace) bumps you over this threshold...no growth!**

This has some interesting implications for structuring an optimal workout. It means **overall** workout speed is important, as well as length of rest between sets and speed of reps within sets!

Pace and Fatigue

You see, the fatigue level of any muscle is constantly changing. Before you start a set, the muscle's fatigue level is low; during the set, it rises; as soon as you finish, it begins to drop as the muscle recovers from the effort. In fact, if you rest long enough, the muscle's fatigue level will drop back to the level from which it began.

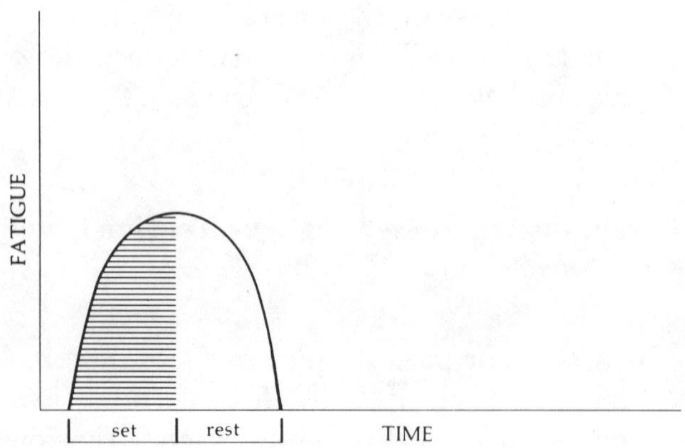

Fig. 2 Fatigue Level During 1 Set

A series of sets, with long rests in between, has a fatigue curve that looks like this:

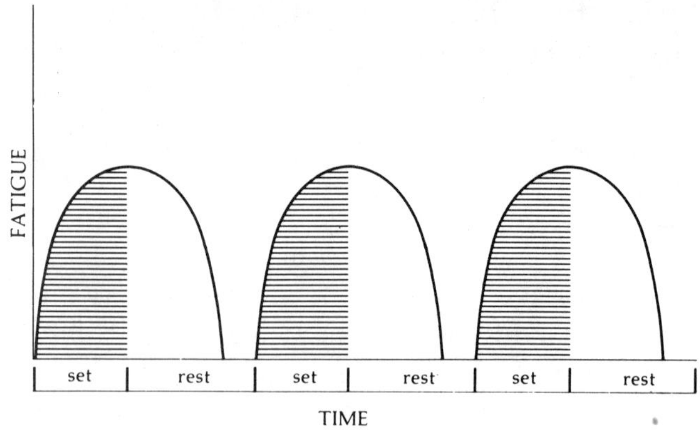

Fig. 3 Fatigue Level During 3 Sets; Long Rests

Notice that as a result of letting the muscle's fatigue level drop so low in between sets, the muscle doesn't get more tired during the second set than during the first, nor more tired during the third than during the second.

Even when you figure in the tension factor, the basic shape of this curve looks the same. The bottom line: no cumulative fatigue effect.

Now, previously, we said a muscle's Fatigue/Tension level must surpass a particular **threshold** for muscle growth to occur. The graph below illustrates why long rests impair progress. Simply, you never cross the threshold.

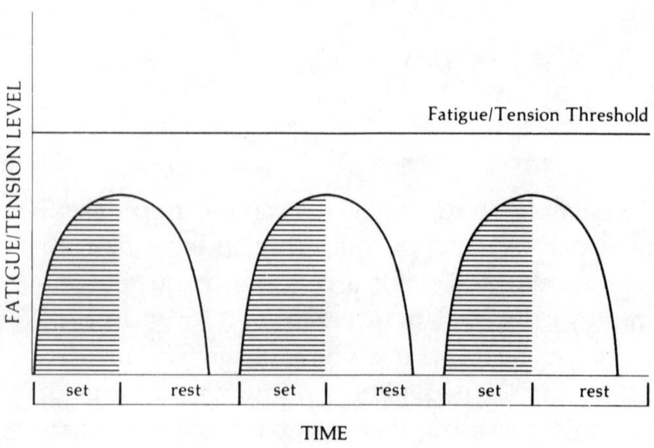

Fig. 4 Fatigue/Tension Threshold

As you shorten the rest time between sets, though, the muscle's fatigue level doesn't have time to drop as far, and you get a stair-step Fatigue/Tension curve that looks like this:

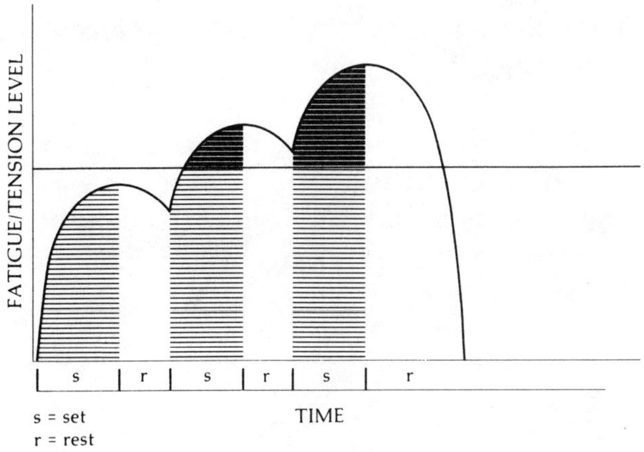

Fig. 5 Fatigue/Tension During 3 Sets; Short Rests

Now the muscle *does* get more tired during the second set than during the first. And during the third set you finally surpass the Fatigue/Tension Threshold. Presto!—*growth.* This is why shorter rests between sets facilitate increases in size and strength.

The same principle applies to rests *between exercises* for the same body part. After doing three or four sets of an exercise, the muscle(s) affected will show some cumulative fatigue level, assuming you are working fast and hard enough. If you rest too long before beginning the next exercise for that same muscle group, the group's fatigue level will drop enough to prevent a cumulative fatigue effect across the different exercises:

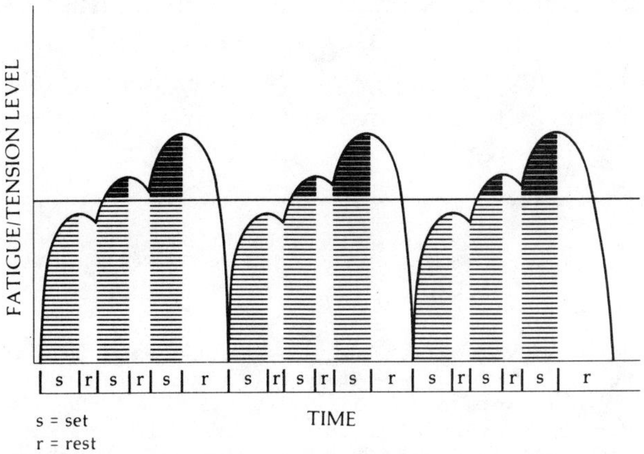

Fig. 6 Fatigue/Tension Level During 3 Exercises; Short Rest Between Sets; Long Rest Between Exercises

"So what?" you may say. "If I've crossed the F/T Threshold during the first exercise for a muscle group, does it really matter that my fatigue level drops before the next?"

Yes! Crossing the F/T is just the beginning of the growth process. Crossing the Threshold—**and staying above it**—is what promotes greater development in less time.

And that's why overall workout speed is important, not just the length of rests between sets or the rep rate. (Also, it's possible you may not cross the F/T Threshold until the second or third exercise for a body part, and may do so then only if you are working fast enough.)

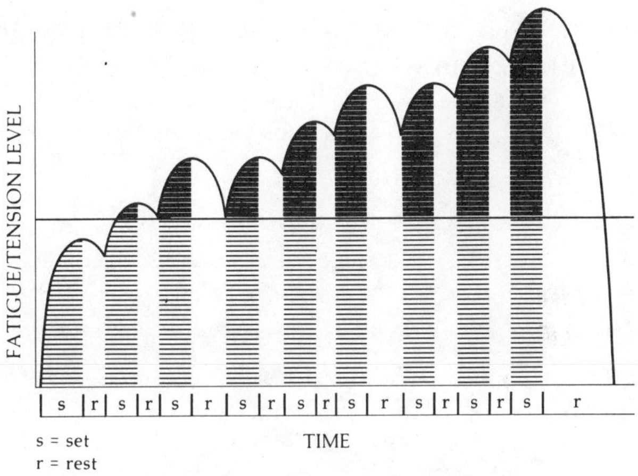

Fig. 7 Fatigue/Tension Level During 3 Exercises; Short Rests Between Sets; Short Rests Between Exercises

Tension

Now let's turn to the question of tension within the Fatigue/Tension concept.

The tension generated within a muscle during exercise depends on four things:

- exercise **form**
- the **load** (amount of weight) you are lifting

- the **leverage** associated with the exercise movement

- and the **mental focus**—the oomph!—you put into your effort.

We will cover *form* in the Exercise Section. For simplicity's sake, let's assume you are going to put an all-out effort into every rep you do; this will keep mental focus constant. So let's take a look at *load* and *leverage.*

Load

The relationship here is simple: Greater load (more weight), more tension...up to a point. As the weight approaches the maximum you can lift, tension within the muscle levels off:

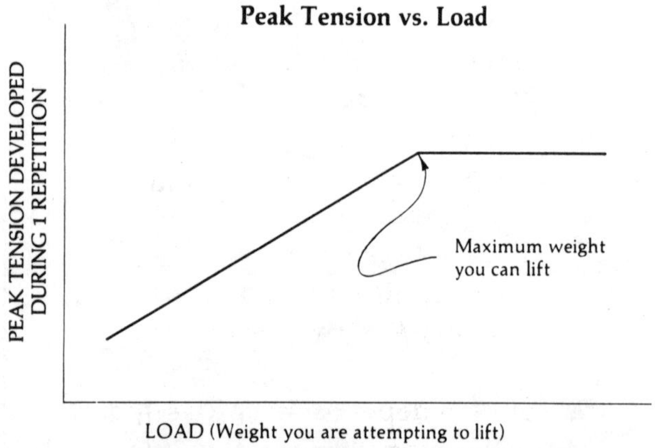

Fig. 8 Peak Tension vs. Load

Now, experience suggests heavy weights are required for building strength and bulk. But keep in mind that weight isn't the only factor involved.

Studies have been done in which a group of athletes/bodybuilders did 3 to 5 sets of various exercises with about 80% of the maximum weight they could lift. Each set consisted of one all-out rep followed by five minutes of rest, then another rep and another rest, and so on until each test subject had performed ten reps total. The athletes followed the regimen three times per week for several months. Then everyone was tested for changes in strength and bulk. The results? Practically no gains! Only a small percentage showed any signs of improvement.

The reason this approach failed is clear in light of the Fatigue/Tension Principle: although tension was kept high, the slow pace kept fatigue low, resulting in a Fatigue/Tension level below the Threshold.*

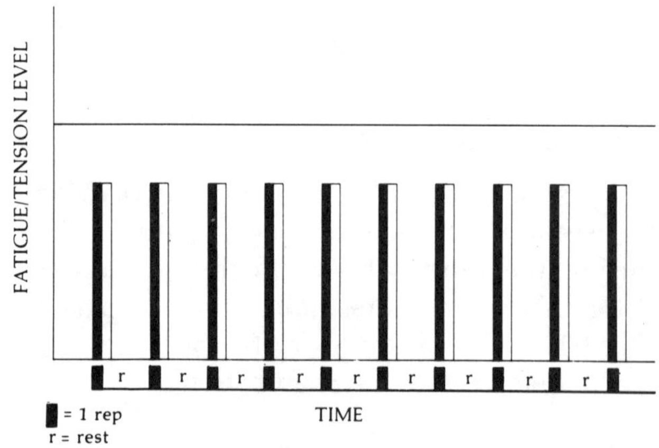

Fig. 9 10 Single Reps; 5 Minute Rests

This is not to say *high load* is unimportant in the growth-inducing formula. Quite the contrary. Using near-maximal poundages has a pronounced effect on a muscle's Fatigue/Tension level. It's just that you must structure your workout to maximize *fatigue*—fast pace, short rests—as well as *tension.* In general, using heavier weights raises the entire F/T curve. It also makes the curve peak at a higher level, because heavier weights increase fatigue as well as tension!

* It *is* possible to generate a tension level sufficient to compensate for an extremely slow pace. This requires using 98% to 100% of the maximum weight you can lift. Power lifters use this sort of workout. We do not recommend this, for two reasons: (1) it puts potentially injurious stress on joints and ligaments; (2) it is not the most effective training program for the combined goals of strength, bulk, and definition.

Here are the curves for the same exercise done at the same pace, first with lighter weights, then with heavier:

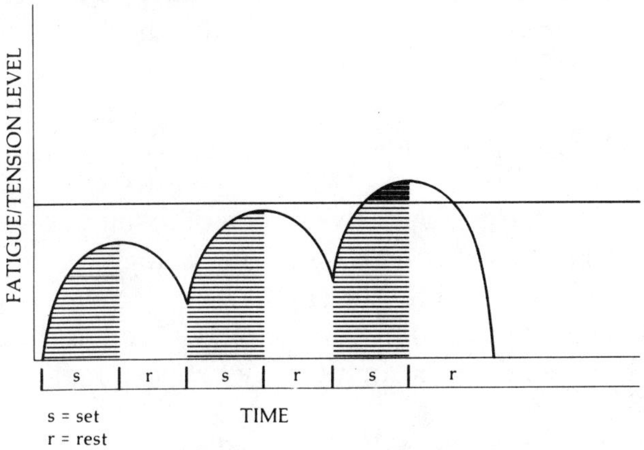

Fig. 10 Fatigue/Tension Level; Light Weight

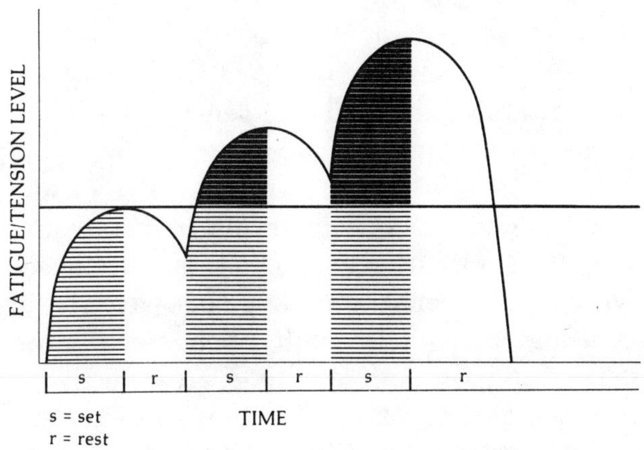

Fig. 11 Fatigue/Tension Level; Heavy Weight

Notice how much steeper the second curve is, and how much sooner it crosses the Fatigue/Tension Threshold.

Leverage

We listed four things that affect the tension generated within a muscle during exercise: form, load, leverage, and mental focus.

Leverage is the most recent of these to be incorporated into workout routines. The last few years have seen the introduction of the "Eccentric Cam" into sophisticated weight training equipment—Nautilus machines, for instance. The Eccentric Cam is an acknowledgement of the fact that the strength of a muscle varies across its range of motion.

Each muscle has its own unique strength curve. A good exercise pits a muscle against resistance that varies in relation to the muscle's strength. This means that for you to *perceive* the resistance as constant, the resistance must vary to match your strength at all points throughout the range of motion.

Through an application of biomechanical principles, it's possible to design exercises that do not involve expensive equipment, but do provide the benefits of variable resistance. This leads to a higher Fatigue/Tension level, and faster growth!

- **Lifting heavy weights does *not* guarantee growth.**
- ***Pace* (number of reps, rep speed, rest length between sets and exercises) combines with *Tension* (dependent on amount of weight lifted) to determine muscular *Fatigue/Tension* level.**
- **Growth depends on surpassing, and staying above, a particular Fatigue/Tension level called the *Fatigue/Tension Threshold.***
- **To be effective, a routine must be structured with *both* Pace and Tension in mind. It will involve heavy poundages and a fast pace that, combined, ensure a stair-step fatigue effect. Also, it will include exercises adjusted to provide resistance closely matched to the leverage of each muscle group.**

SPECIAL FATIGUE/TENSION CONSIDERATIONS FOR TRAINING CALVES

Perhaps the most profound ability of living organisms (like humans) is adaptation. Indeed, muscle growth is exactly that—muscle adaptation to stress.

The kind of adaptive response you get depends on the kind of stress you put on the organism. If you force a muscle to act against incredible amounts of resistance (such as doing a Bench Press with a bunch of 45's packed on each end of the bar), the muscle develops greater contractile power. If, on the other hand, you force a muscle to contract hundreds upon hundreds of times without resting, it develops greater endurance.

That is exactly what constant walking, running, and standing have done to your calves: given them *excellent* endurance.

One consequence of that endurance is a greater recovery ability compared with many other skeletal muscles. If we take the graph we've been using over the last few pages as illustrating the exercise/recovery cycle of your "average" muscle—your biceps, say—then a similar graph for the calves would look like this:

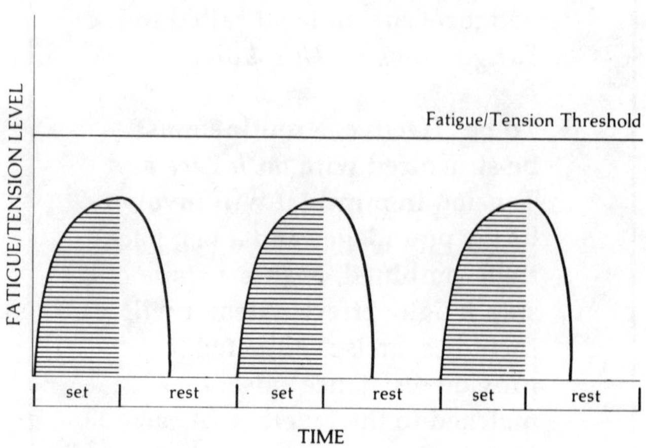

Fig. 12 Fatigue/Tension Level During 3 Sets of a Calf Exercise

The sharp fall-off over the part of the graph labeled *rest* represents the fact that, after exertion, the calves' fatigue level drops much more quickly than many other muscles' fatigue levels. In other words, they recover faster.

Consequences for training?

For starters, the calves' incredible endurance makes it difficult to achieve a high fatigue level during sets. In effect, they're constantly "recovering" from your efforts, even during the brief decrease in intensity between reps.

Second, their endurance makes it difficult to maintain a high fatigue level over the course of several sets or exercises, because, even during a short rest, they recover almost completely. That means it's hard to surpass and remain above the Fatigue/Tension Threshold necessary for growth.

The usual methods of trying to get around the calves' endurance "problem" are doing sets with phenomenal amounts of weight (increasing *tension*), or with phenomenal numbers of reps. Both methods are effective at increasing the calves' Fatigue/Tension level during sets, although high weight/low reps is clearly more time-efficient.

The key words in that last sentence are "during sets." Remember, stimulating growth requires elevating a muscle's fatigue level above the Fatigue/Tension Threshold and maintaining it there. **Neither method addresses keeping the calves' fatigue level high *across sets.***

And that opens the door to a major improvement in calf training technique.

By substituting a low-intensity calf exercise for the rest periods between sets of high-intensity work, it's possible to achieve the desired stair-step Fatigue/Tension level across sets. And that—means growth!

- **The calves have better endurance, and thus greater recovery ability, than many other skeletal muscles.**

- **Problem: This greater recovery ability makes it difficult to achieve and maintain a high calf Fatigue/Tension level across sets or exercises.**

- **Solution: Replace rests between high-intensity sets with a low-intensity exercise designed to allow only partial recovery.**

INTERDEPENDENCY OF MUSCLE GROUPS

Research has demonstrated there is *one particular sequence* of a given series of exercises that affords maximum benefit to all muscles involved. This sequence makes each of the exercises more effective than those same exercises performed in random order. This optimal sequence is partly determined by a principle called the **Interdependency of Muscle Groups**, which states that, in the performance of certain movements, some muscles depend on others. Here's how this applies to your calves....

The two big muscles in the back of the calf—the gastrocnemius and soleus—are both plantar flexors. That is, they both act to bend the ankle down.

You can't exercise the gastroc without calling the soleus into play because of the interdependency of these two muscle groups. You can, however, exercise the soleus separately by employing a simple technique we will discuss in the exercise section.

To work the Soleus, you use:

SOLEUS

To work the Gastrocnemius, you use:

GASTROCNEMIUS + SOLEUS

Notice the soleus plays a role in the work you do for both muscles. As a result, if you tire the soleus first, it becomes the weak link in the chain, limiting the amount of gastroc work you can do. **The formula for optimum effectiveness calls for working the gastroc first.** That way you can burn out the gastroc completely, then work the soleus to its limit with exercises that focus on it.

As a bonus, once the soleus is tired from gastroc work, it won't need to be pushed as hard to get a good workout.

We can make a similar argument for doing planter flexor/dorsiflexor work before pronator/supinator work. Pronators and supinators are involved in *stabilizing* your ankles (holding them in place) when you do plantar flexor and dorsiflexor exercises. The pronators and supinators, however, can also be called upon directly with exercises that concentrate on them. In other words...

To work the Pronators or Supinators, you use:

PRONATORS OR SUPINATORS

To work the Plantar Flexors or Dorsiflexors, you use:

PLANTAR FLEXORS OR DORSIFLEXORS
+
PRONATORS AND SUPINATORS

If you were to work the pronators and supinators before doing dorsiflexor work, you might find yourself with unstable ankles trying to do a Donkey Calf Raise with a two-hundred pound partner on your back!

Pronator/supinator exercises should *follow* plantar flexor/dorsiflexor exercises.

- **Exercise order, dictated by the Interdependency of Muscle Groups, can dramatically improve exercise efficiency.**
- **For calves, this means:**
  - ❑ **gastroc exercises should preceed soleus exercises**
  - ❑ **plantar flexor/dorsiflexor exercises should preceed pronator/supinator exercises**

FUNCTIONAL STRENGTH AND ISOLATION

The final concept we will consider that has an impact on exercise order is the distinction between **functional strength** exercises and **isolation** exercises.

Functional strength refers to the ability to apply strength, developed through exercise, in daily life.

Not surprisingly, the exercises most effective at developing functional strength are those most resembling movements that occur in daily life. A Squat, for example, is a lot like lifting a heavy box off the floor. Likewise, a Bench Press resembles pushing a couch around your living room; a Standing Bicep Curl is like picking up a package.

What **functional strength exercises** have in common is that they involve the body as a whole. They make heavy demands, not only on the target muscle group (e.g. the pecs during a Bench Press), but also on many supporting muscles which must all work together to generate the required movement. In contrast, *isolation* exercises make substantially less-intense demands on supporting muscles.

Example:

When doing Donkey Calf Raises (a functional strength calf exercise), your thighs, glutes, back, abs, and even arms have to work hard to keep your body in position on the calf block (to *stabilize* it). They provide a solid foundation from which your plantar flexors can act to lift your body.

In contrast, when doing Seated Calf Raises (an isolation calf exercise), the machine takes care of most the stabilizing. Most of the actual work is done by the target muscle group—the soleus.

Two kinds of exercises, two different effects.

Functional strength exercises and the kind of strength they develop are important for overall health and effectiveness in day-to-day physical activity. **Also, they have been shown to stimulate growth throughout the body, not just in the target muscle group.** In other words, functional strength exercises are *synergistic*—do them, and your entire routine becomes more effective!

Isolation exercises, on the other hand, are important for focusing on specific muscle groups or parts of specific muscle groups. **Done alone, not in combination with FSE's, they produce a kind of strength—an *isolated* strength—which is *not* useful in day-to-day life.**

The bottom line: a balanced workout includes both.

However, **functional strength exercises should preceed isolation exercises**, because...

FSE's are most effective when performed with heavy weights—and in the interest of safety, it's better to do high-poundage exercises before you tire the supporting muscles for a body part. Doing FSE's with heavy weights maximizes the involved muscles' Fatigue/Tension levels, tires the target muscle group sufficiently for later isolation exercises to have maximum effect, and puts sufficient stress on the ligaments to strengthen them.

That last point is very important. Only a substantial overload—such as the kind you get doing FSE's with heavy weight—puts sufficient stress on your musculoskeletal system to strengthen ligaments and thicken bones.*

- **Functional strength exercises closely match the ways you use interdependent muscles in everyday life.**
- **FSE's stimulate growth throughout the body, not just in the target muscle group.**
- **Isolation exercises are important for focusing on specific muscle groups or parts of specific muscle groups.**
- **Functional strength exercises should preceed isolation exercises.**

* For a more detailed discussion of functional and isolation exercises, see the *Exercise Sequence* chapter of our book, **Secrets of Advanced Bodybuilders.**

REVIEW

We now have the information necessary to begin structuring an effective calf program. Before getting down to the specifics of the exercises, though, let's take a moment to review.

Anatomy

- The calves are responsible for two pairs of opposing ankle movements:
  - ❑ plantar flexion / dorsiflexion
  - ❑ pronation / supination
- Each movement is the result of several calf muscles working together in a **muscle group**.
- In our quest for mass and/or strength, we will be working for balanced development of the opposing muscle groups. This will increase functional strength, footwork speed, and ankle stability. It will also decrease risk of ankle injury.

Fatigue/Tension Principle

- Lifting heavy weights does *not* guarantee growth.
- **Pace** (rep speed, rest length between sets and exercises) combines with **tension** (dependent on amount of weight lifted) to determine muscular **Fatigue/Tension** level.
- Growth depends on surpassing and staying above a particular Fatigue/Tension level called the **Fatigue/Tension Threshold**.
- To be effective, a routine must be structured with *both* pace and tension in mind. It will involve heavy poundages and a fast pace that, combined, ensure a stair-step fatigue effect. Also, it will include exercises adjusted to provide resistance closely matched to the leverage of each muscle group.

Continued...

Special Fatigue/Tension Considerations for Training Calves

- The calves have better endurance than many other skeletal muscles, and thus recover faster.
- This faster recovery makes it difficult to achieve and maintain a high calf fatigue level across sets or exercises.
- To circumvent this problem, we will replace rests between high-intensity sets with a low-intensity exercise designed to allow only partial recovery.

Interdependency of Muscle Groups

- Exercise order, dictated by the Interdependency of Muscle Groups, can dramatically improve exercise efficiency.

  For calves, this means:

  - ❑ gastroc exercises will preceed soleus exercises
  - ❑ plantar flexor/dorsiflexor exercises will preceed pronator/supinator exercises

Functional Strength

- Functional strength exercises closely match the ways you use interdependent muscles in everyday life.
- FSE's stimulate growth throughout the body, not just in the target muscle group.
- Isolation exercises are important for focusing on specific muscle groups or parts of specific muscle groups.
- Functional strength exercises will preceed isolation exercises.

☆ ☆ ☆

PROGRAM SECTION

THE EXERCISES

The exercises illustrated in this section are the building blocks of the **Maximum Calves** routines. You're probably familiar with some of them. However, the exercise descriptions contain subtleties of form specific to this course. **It's these details, *along with the specific sequence and timing listed in the program section*,** that make **Maximum Calves** such an effective conditioning tool.

THE CALF BLOCK

Many calf exercises involve a block. Ideally, it should:

- be four to six inches high (to allow a full stretch)
- have a slightly-rounded front edge (to make levering up and down on its edge more comfortable)
- not be slippery (glue a rubber strip to the part your feet will touch, if need be)
- be rock stable.

Best is the steps on a Nautilus Calf Machine (Fig. 13-a). Second best is a block specifically designed for calf work (Fig. 13-b). These usually have some sort of frame on the bottom to ensure stability, and a non-skid strip—the kind you find on the bottom of hotel room shower stalls—on one edge to prevent your slipping off. Third best is a stair. Least preferable, but adequate if you have no other options, is a 6" x 12" wood block (Fig. 13-c).

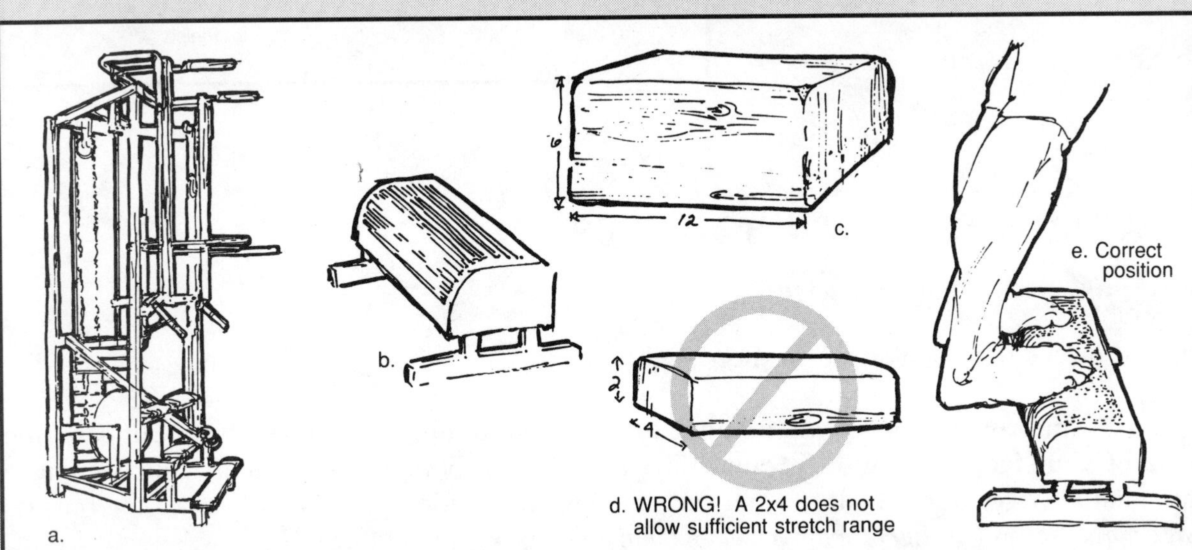

Fig. 13

A two-by-four is not satisfactory, as it does not allow sufficient stretch range (Fig. 13-d).

When standing on the block, make sure the ball of your foot is just over the edge (Fig. 13-e). Standing too far forward or back causes the ankle to hinge unnaturally, putting unnecessary, and possibly injurious, stress on it.

WARMUP #1 — STANDING TOE PULL-BACKS

prime mover: dorsiflexors

Stand on the floor with your feet shoulder-width apart, toes pointing forward, knees bent, body inclined forward slightly (Fig. 14-a). (If you ski, this is your standard push-off position.)

Dorsiflex—pull the front of your foot up toward your shin—allowing your knees to straighten slightly (Fig. 14-b). Feel for the squeeze in your anterior tibialis muscles (along the front of your shins), then lower your toes to the ground and repeat. Rate should be about one rep per second.

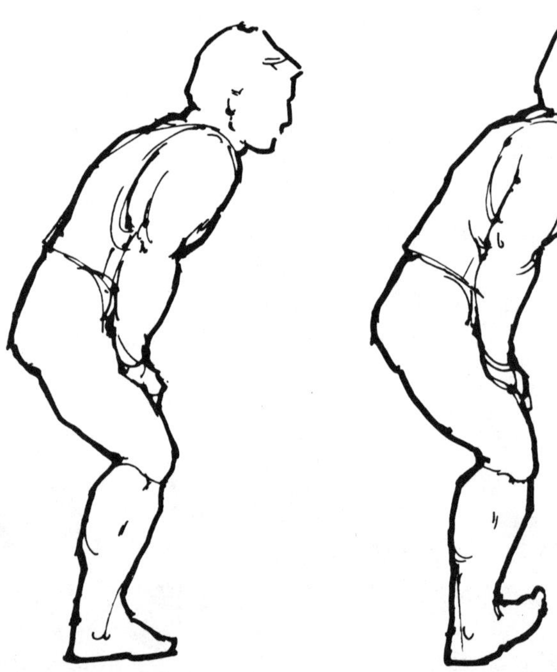

a. Start b. Finish

Fig. 14

WARMUP #2 — CALF BOUNCES

prime mover: plantar flexors

Stand on the floor on your toes, knees slightly bent.

Bounce quickly up and down **without allowing your heels to touch the ground or the balls of your feet to leave the ground** (Fig. 15). As you bounce, slowly shift your weight to the outside edges of the balls of your feet, then to the inside edges, then back to the outside edges, and so on (see *Important Technique Point #1* in box on next page).

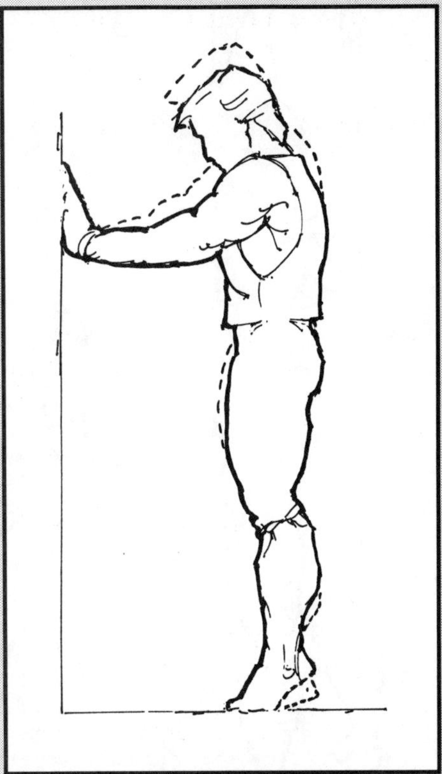

Fig. 15

Continue bouncing **without slowing** for 45 seconds to one minute. Rate: about 15 bounces per 5 seconds.

If you need help maintaining your balance, rest your hands against a wall during the exercise.

IMPORTANT TECHNIQUE POINT #1

Shifting Emphasis from Outer to Inner Plantar Flexor Heads

The "shifting" referred to in the plantar flexor warmup description involves very little motion—just a slight change in the degree of pronation/supination at the ankles. (The balls of your feet remain flat on the floor or block.) **However, the change in mechanical stress on the calves is severe, shifting the emphasis from outer head of soleus and gastrocnemius to inner head.** Accomplishing that change plays an important role in the effectiveness of the **Maximum Calves** routines, and we will be using the technique during many of the exercises.

The more standard method of shifting emphasis from outer to inner calf—doing some exercises with toes pointed out, then some with toes pointed in—places considerably more stress on ankle and knee joints. Since an alternate, and equally effective, method for accomplishing that goal exists, we strongly recommend against using toe out/toe in.

SINGLE-LEG CALF RAISES

prime mover: plantar flexors

Stand on the block on your right foot, supporting yourself against the wall. **Don't bring your left foot behind your right; this puts most of the emphasis of the exercise on the outer plantar flexors, and makes it difficult to shift that emphasis anywhere else.**

Part 1.

With your supporting leg **straight**—knee locked or bent very, very slightly (see insert #1)—lower yourself as far as possible, feeling for the stretch (Fig. 16-a).

Then push up with your weight on the outer edge of your foot, focusing the stress on the outer head of the plantar flexor group (Fig. 16-b). Use two thrusts: The first should take you through about 80% of your range of motion; the second should take you as far as you can go. Hold for a second at peak, then lower and repeat.

After the number of reps indicated in the Routines Section, shift the emphasis from outer to inner head by changing your weight distribution and the degree of pronation at your ankle (Fig. 16-c,d). Remember—the shift of emphasis is mostly a matter of "feel." The actual movement at your ankle is slight.

Part 2.

Without stopping, repeat Part 1 with your knee bent and your body hunched over slightly (see insert #2, and Fig. 16-e,f,g,h). The significance of this seemingly insignificant position change is explained in the box on page 20 labeled *Important Technique Point #2* .

Repeat the entire exercise using your other leg.

If you need a greater overload to achieve a burn, both Parts 1 & 2 can be performed with a dumbell held in the same-side hand (e.g. if you're pushing with right leg, hold weight in right hand—Fig. 16-i). Simple reason here—you need the other hand to support yourself.

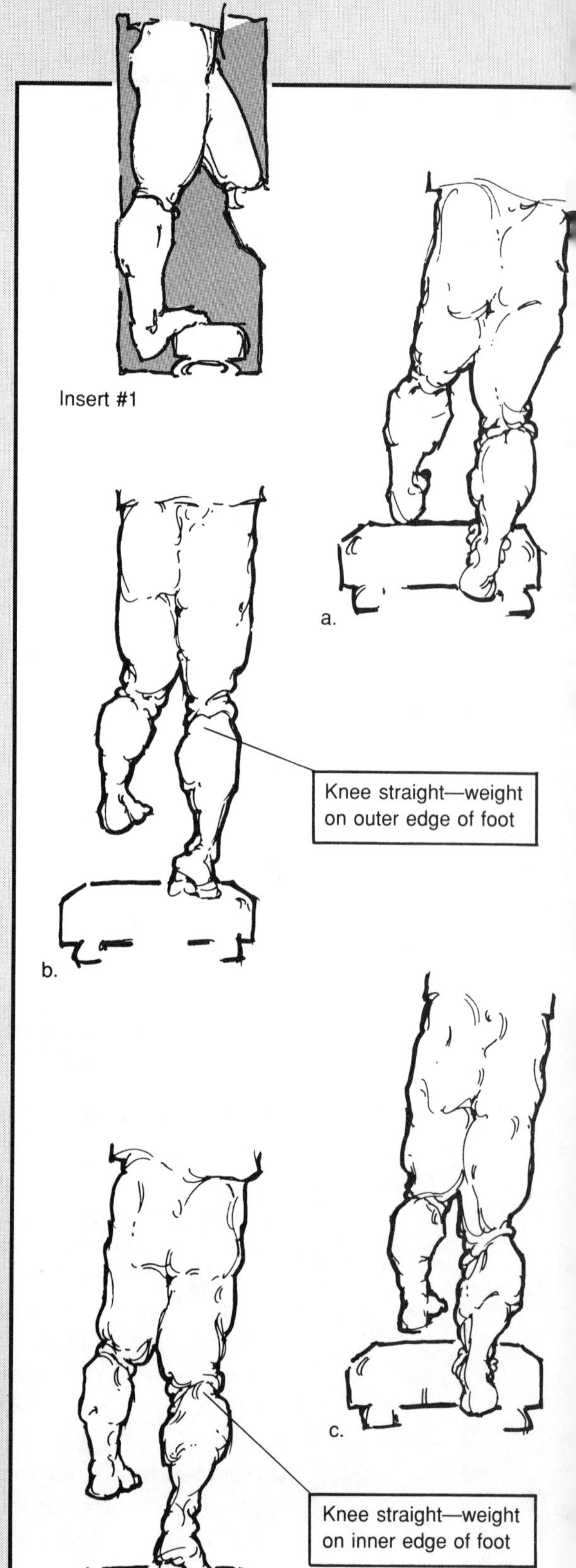

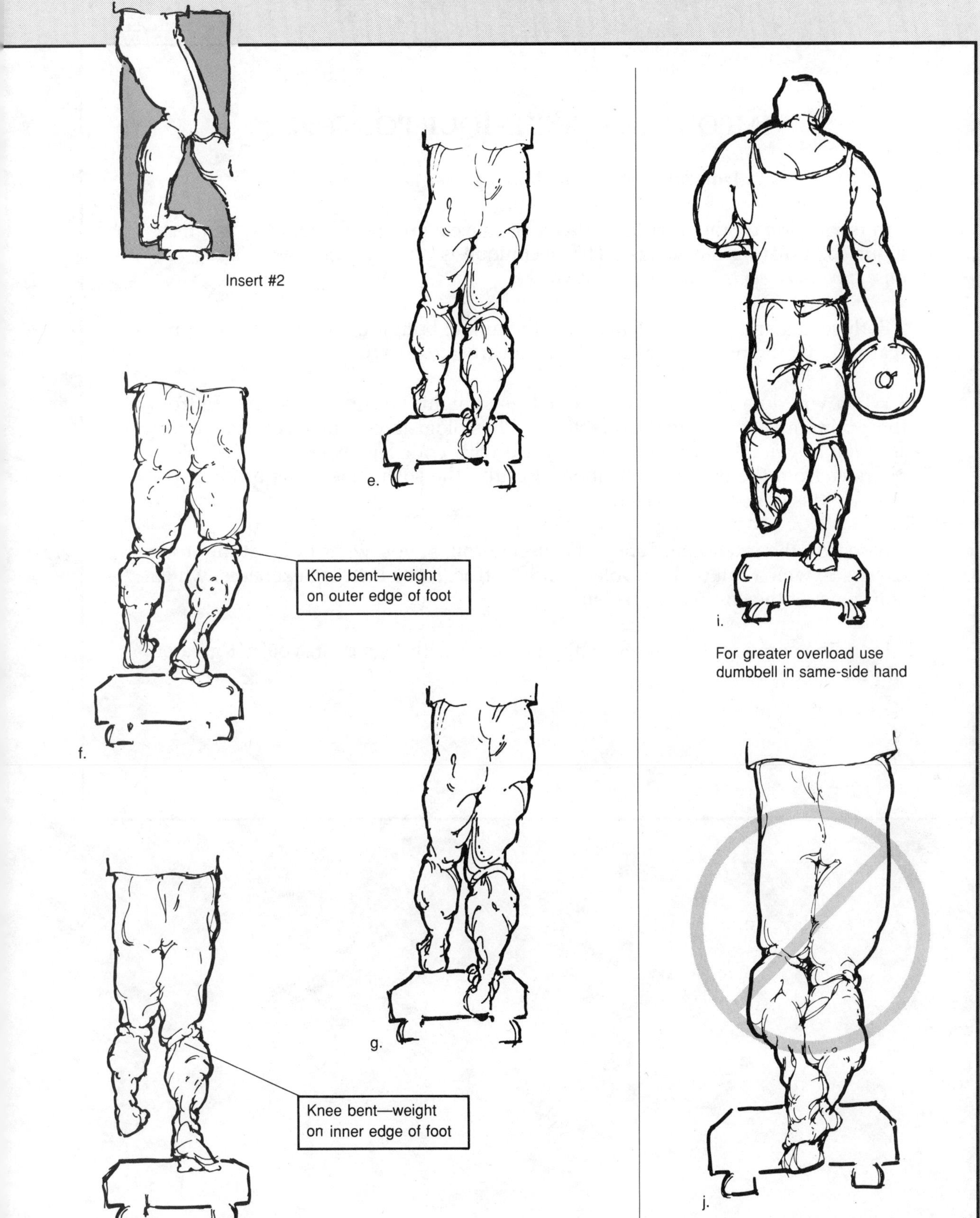
Insert #2
e.
Knee bent—weight on outer edge of foot
f.
g.
Knee bent—weight on inner edge of foot
h.
i.
For greater overload use dumbbell in same-side hand
j.
WRONG! Don't cross one foot behind the other

Fig. 16

IMPORTANT TECHNIQUE POINT #2

Isolating the Soleus During Plantar Flexion

In the section on the interdependency of muscle groups, we alluded to a technique for isolating the soleus. That technique is *bending your knees during calf-raise-type movements*. Here's why it works:

Both soleus and gastroc plantar flex the ankle; both are located on the upper rear calf. Of the two, however, only the gastroc crosses the knee joint.

When you do a calf raise with your legs straight, both muscles operate from the optimum position for contraction. Physiologists call this position *resting stretched length*. When you do a calf raise with your legs bent, only the soleus operates from the optimum position. Result: the soleus takes the brunt of the stress and is effectively isolated.

Based on the interdependency of muscle groups, you want to do straight leg exercises, which call on both soleus and gastroc, *before* bent leg exercises, which shift most of the stress to the soleus.

By doing some reps with legs straight, some with legs bent, you get greater, more even development!

DONKEY OR NAUTILUS CALF RAISES

prime mover: plantar flexors

Block stability is very important during this exercise.

Position the block so you can stand on its edge. Bend at the waist, and support yourself on a horizontal bar or table at just above waist height, as illustrated below (Fig. 17-a,b). Have a partner straddle your back. Your partner's weight should be centered as directly above your hips as possible.

Now, go through the entire sequence described under Single-Leg Calf Raises:

- Begin with legs straight (insert #1, next page).
- Using the two-step thrust motion, push up with the weight on the outer edges of your feet (Fig. 18-a,b). Hold for a second at peak before beginning the next rep.
- Do the number of reps specified in the program section.
- **Without stopping**, shift your weight from the outer to the inner edges of your feet to shift focus from outer to inner head of the plantar flexors (Fig. 18-c,d).
- Complete the number of reps specified in the program section.
- **Without stopping**, repeat the entire sequence with legs bent (insert #2, Fig. 18-e,f,g,h).

If you have a Nautilus Calf Machine available to you, you can perform the exercise without a partner (Fig. 17-c). However, the movement is slightly less effective this way because the chain stabilizes you, diminishing the "functional strength" aspect of the exercise.

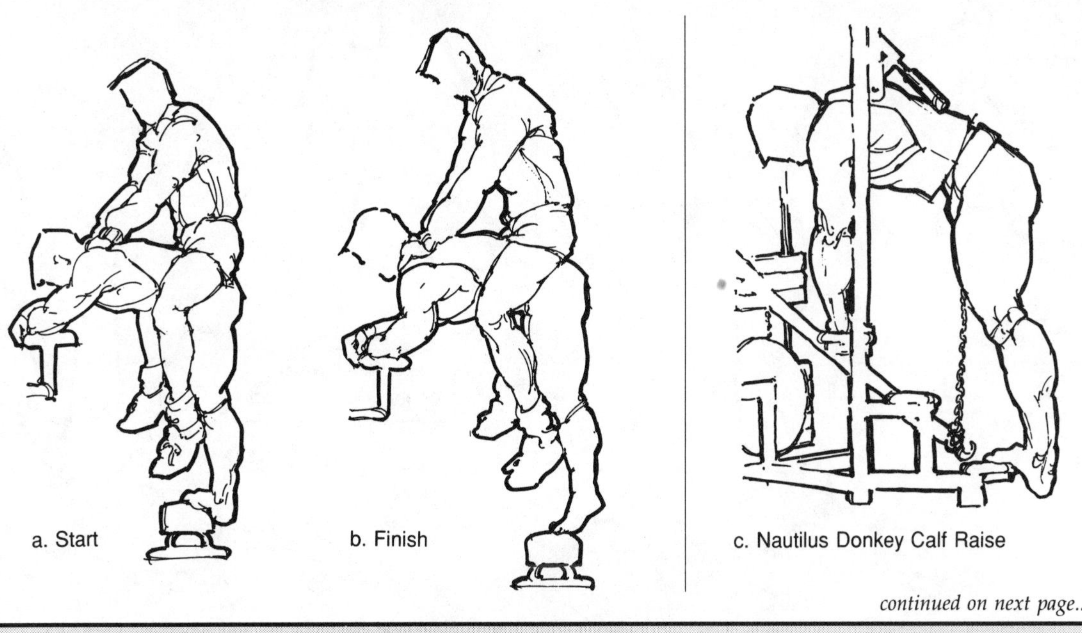

a. Start

b. Finish

c. Nautilus Donkey Calf Raise

continued on next page...

Fig. 17

FOOT POSITIONS FOR DONKEY CALF RAISES

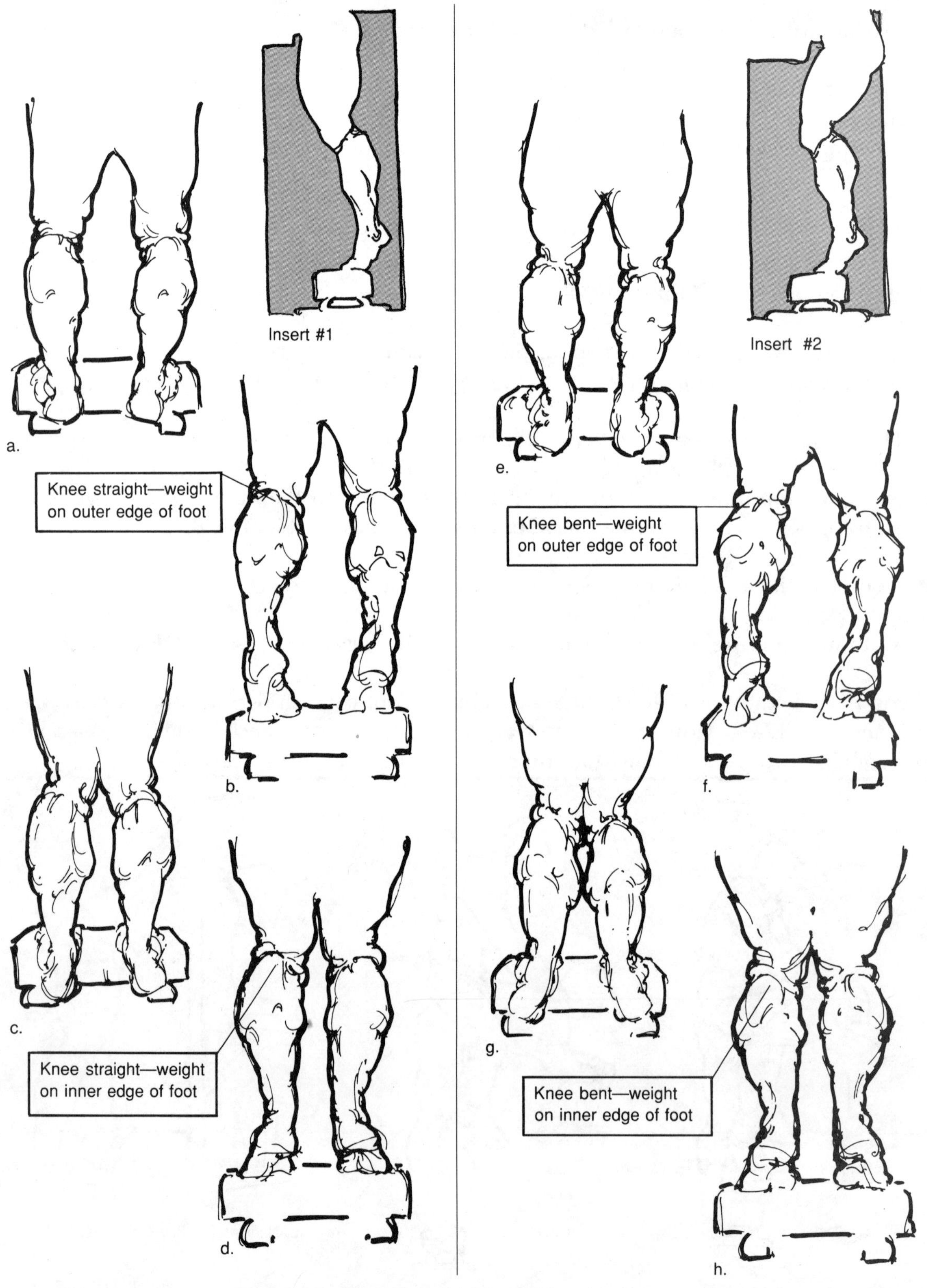

Fig. 18

CALF ROCK-UPS

prime mover: plantar flexors

This is the "low-intensity" movement referred to in the Fatigue/Tension section. It will be used at various points within the routines to maintain a high fatigue level in the plantar flexors while allowing sufficient recovery so you can continue. **It is not intended to function as an exercise in its own right, and will not feel like much done apart from the routines.**

Squat, supporting yourself on the balls of your feet, using a vertical bar for balance (Fig. 19-a). Lean forward slightly. Your heels should not be touching the ground.

Quickly rock up onto the balls of your feet, raising your heels as high as possible. Keep your body relaxed except for the plantar flexors (Fig. 19-b). Lower and repeat. Rate: about 8 bounces per 5 seconds. Your heels should not touch the ground at any time during the exercise.

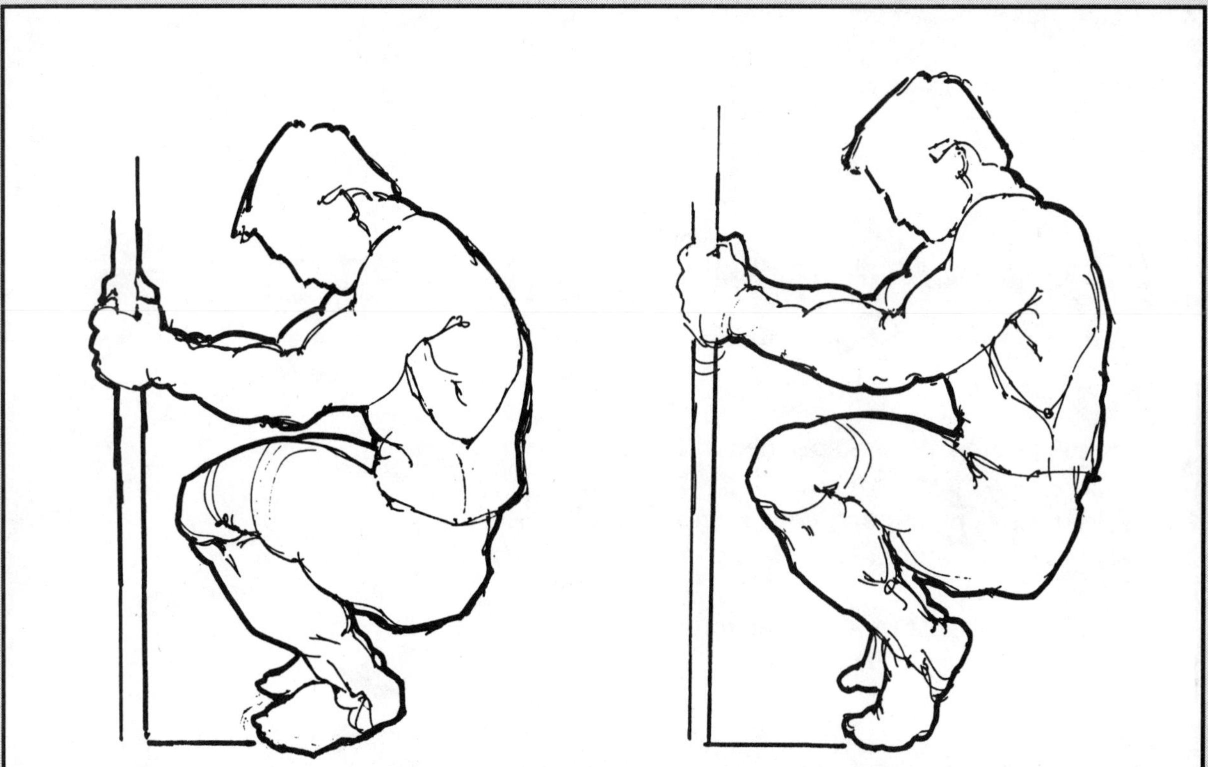

a. Start

b. Finish

Fig. 19

STANDING CALF RAISES

prime mover: plantar flexors

Often recommended as the mainstay of calf programs, this exercise actually functions better as an isolation or supplementary exercise, for two reasons:

- The bars which transfer the resistance to your shoulders also stabilize you, limiting the functional strength aspect of the exercise.
- The machine places considerable stress on the spine. Doing the exercise late in the routine when your calves are already tired allows you to use less weight (thus placing less stress on the spine) and still achieve the same Fatigue/Tension level.

Put an amount of weight on the stack that will barely allow you to complete the indicated number of reps. Starting with your knees bent and **your body upright**, position your shoulders against the weight bars, and extend your knees to get into position (Fig. 20-a,b). Starting out bent at the waist and then straightening the torso to get into position puts potentially injurious stress on your lower back.

Perform the exercise as follows:

First Set

- Begin with legs straight (Fig. 21, insert #1).
- Using the two-step thrust motion, push up with the weight on the outer edges of your feet (Fig. 21-a,b). Hold for a second at peak before beginning the next rep.
- Do the number of reps specified in the program section.
- Without stopping, **bend your knees** (Fig. 21, insert #2) and **continue** to push up with the weight on the outer edges of your feet (Fig. 21-c,d).
- Do the number of reps specified in the program section.

Next Set

- Begin with legs straight (Fig. 21, insert #3).
- Using the two-step thrust motion, push up with the weight on the *inner* edges of your feet (Fig. 21-e,f). Hold for a second at peak before beginning the next rep.
- Do the number of reps specified in the program section.
- Without stopping, **bend your knees** (Fig. 21, insert #4) and *continue* to push up with the weight on the *inner* edges of your feet (Fig. 21-g,h).
- Do the number of reps specified in the program section.

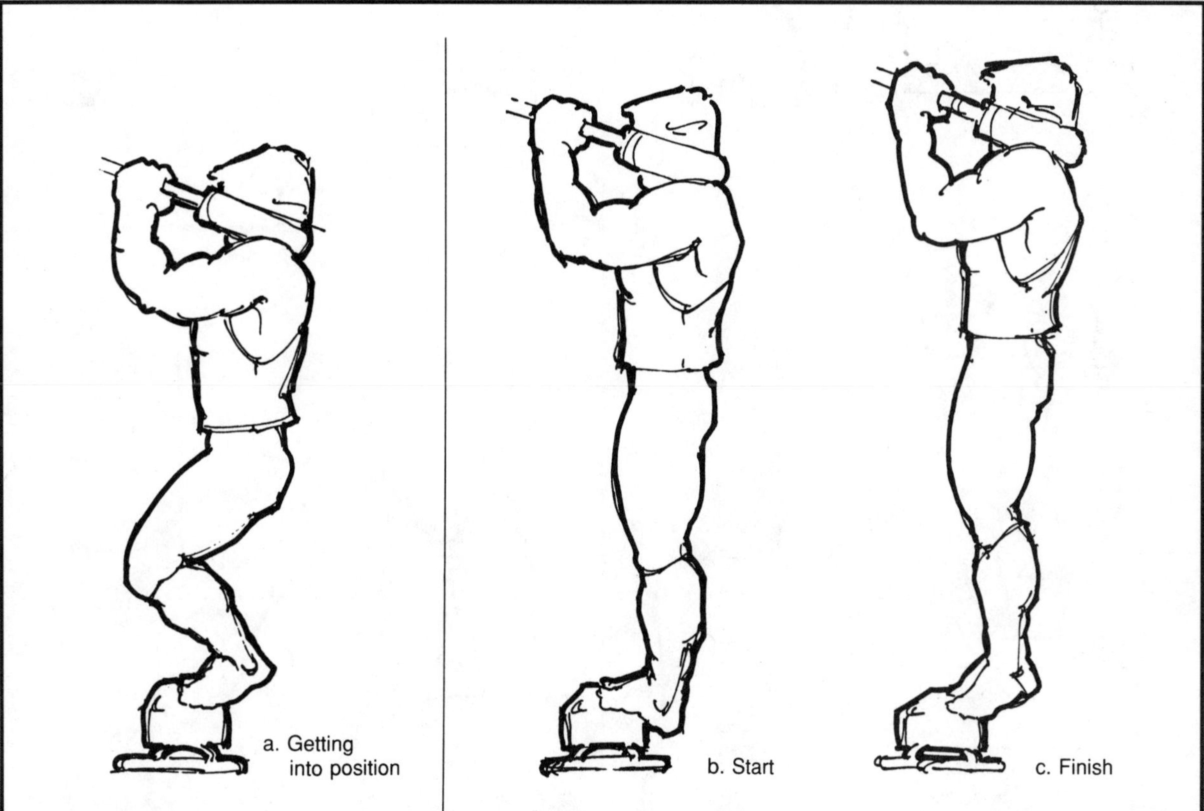

continued on next page...

Fig. 20

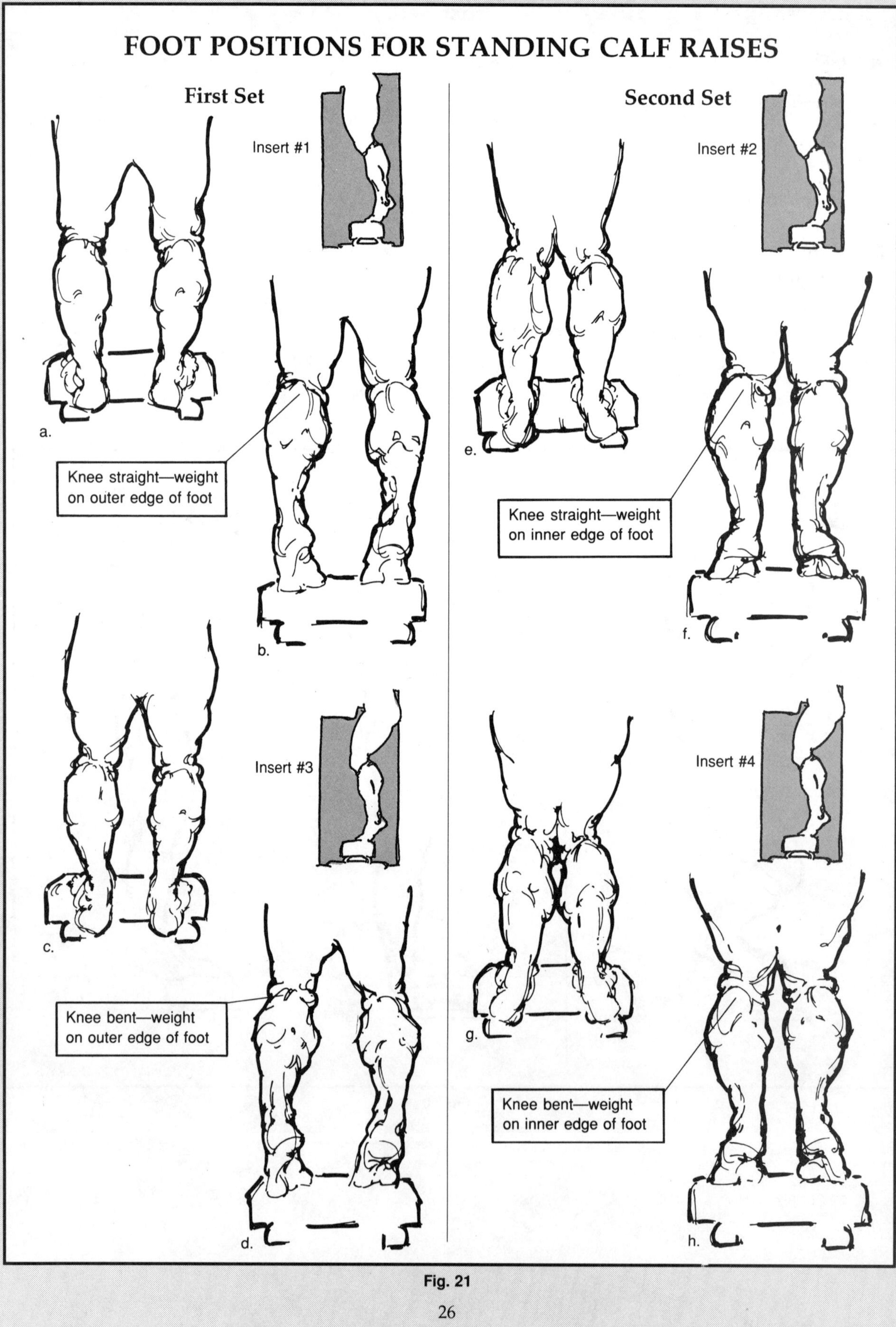
FOOT POSITIONS FOR STANDING CALF RAISES
First Set
Insert #1
a.
Knee straight—weight on outer edge of foot
b.
Insert #3
c.
Knee bent—weight on outer edge of foot
d.
Second Set
Insert #2
e.
Knee straight—weight on inner edge of foot
f.
Insert #4
g.
Knee bent—weight on inner edge of foot
h.

Fig. 21

SEATED CALF RAISES

prime mover: plantar flexors

This exercise isolates the calves more effectively than any other exercise. For the reasons explained in the box on page 20, it is more effective at the end of a calf workout than at the beginning.

Unless otherwise noted in the Routines Section, do outer and inner plantar flexor heads in alternate sets.

The basic movement involves performing calf raises in a seated position. There are three different equipment setups you can use to do this.

First is the standard Seated Calf Raise Machine (Fig. 22-a,b). If you use this machine, make sure you don't sit so far forward that the angle at your knee is less than 90 degrees (Fig. 22-c).

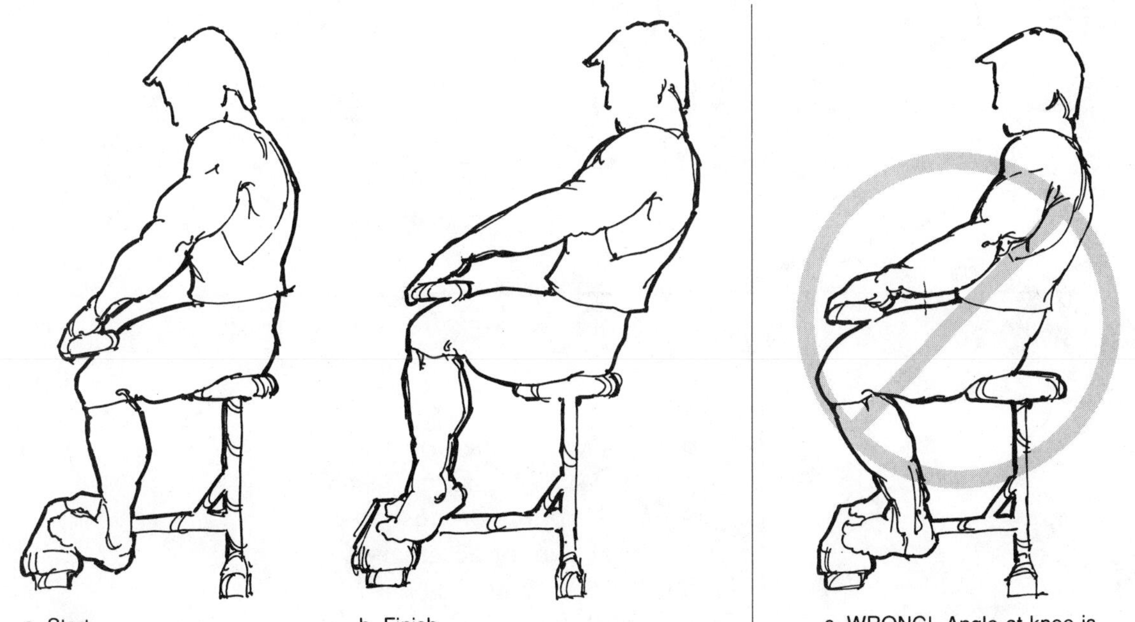

a. Start

b. Finish

c. WRONG! Angle at knee is less than 90 degrees

Fig. 22

Second is the Bench Press on a Universal gym. You will need a partner to help you get into position for this version.

Lie on the bench, face down, knees bent. Have your partner lift the bar. Position the balls of your feet under the bar, and have your partner **slowly** lower it onto your feet (Fig. 23-a). Press to full extension using the two-step thrust (Fig. 23-b,c); hold for a second, then lower the bar as far as possible, feeling for the stretch in your plantar flexors. Repeat.

Make sure your partner is standing by to lift the weight off your feet when you finish the set.

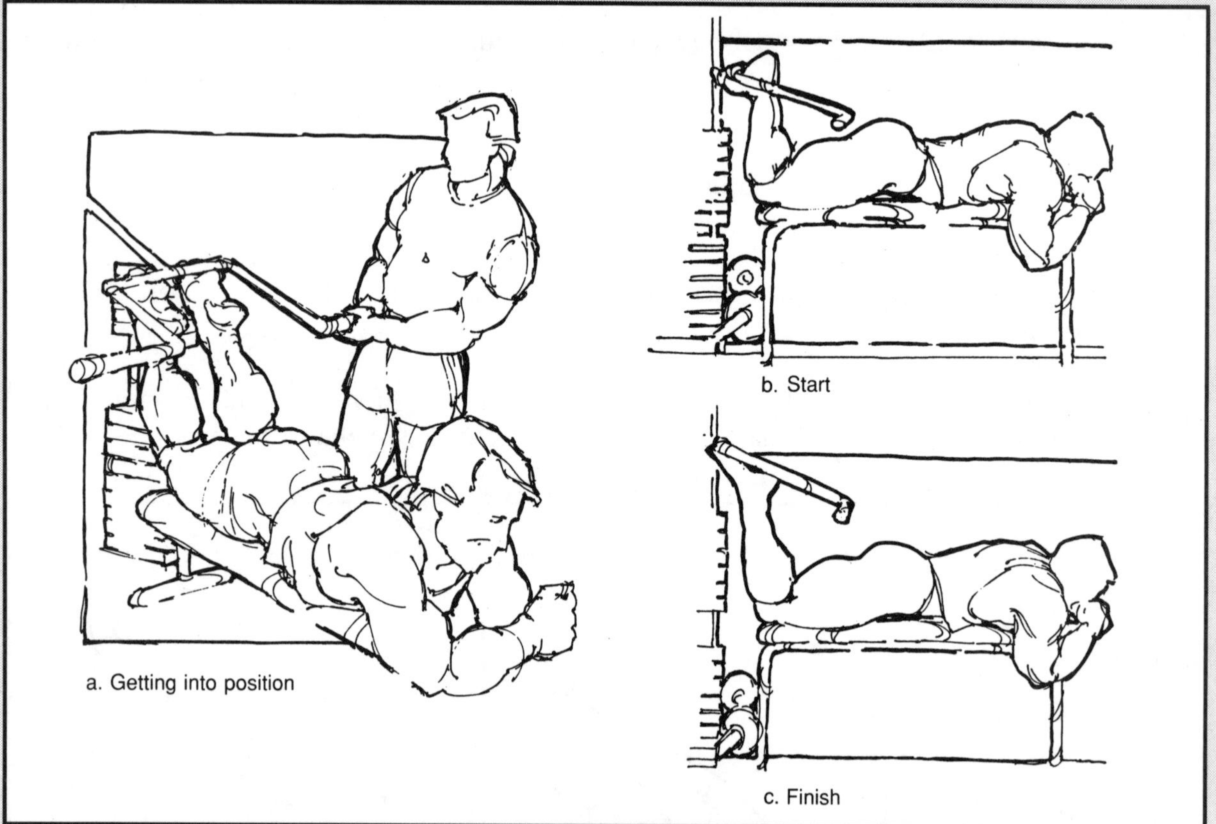

a. Getting into position

b. Start

c. Finish

Fig. 23

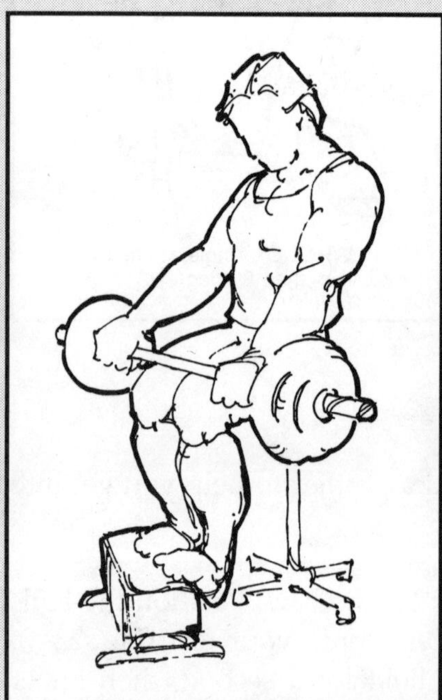

Fig. 24

Finally, you can simply place a barbell across a pad on your lap (Fig. 24). This is the least preferable option, because the amount of weight necessary to overload the plantar flexors will rapidly exceed what you can comfortably—and safely—position on your lap. However, if you have no other choice, this setup will do for a start.

SEATED TOE PULL-BACKS

prime mover: dorsiflexors

This move can be performed using any of three resistance devices: the *dard*, iron boot, or rubber strap.

Using the *Dard*

The *dard* (Fig. 25-a) is specifically designed for this exercise, and is your best equipment choice. (Unfortunately, you won't find one lying around in every gym.†) It allows you to work both legs at once, decreasing workout time and improving mechanical stability.

Begin by sitting on a straight bench, both legs straight, feet extending off the end. Position the *dard* as shown in Figure 25-b below. Slowly pull your feet back as far as possible, lifting the weight (Fig. 25-c). Pull evenly with both feet.

Hold for one second, then lower to starting position. Feel for maximum stretch in the dorsiflexors, especially the anterior tibialis muscles along your shins.

Repeat.

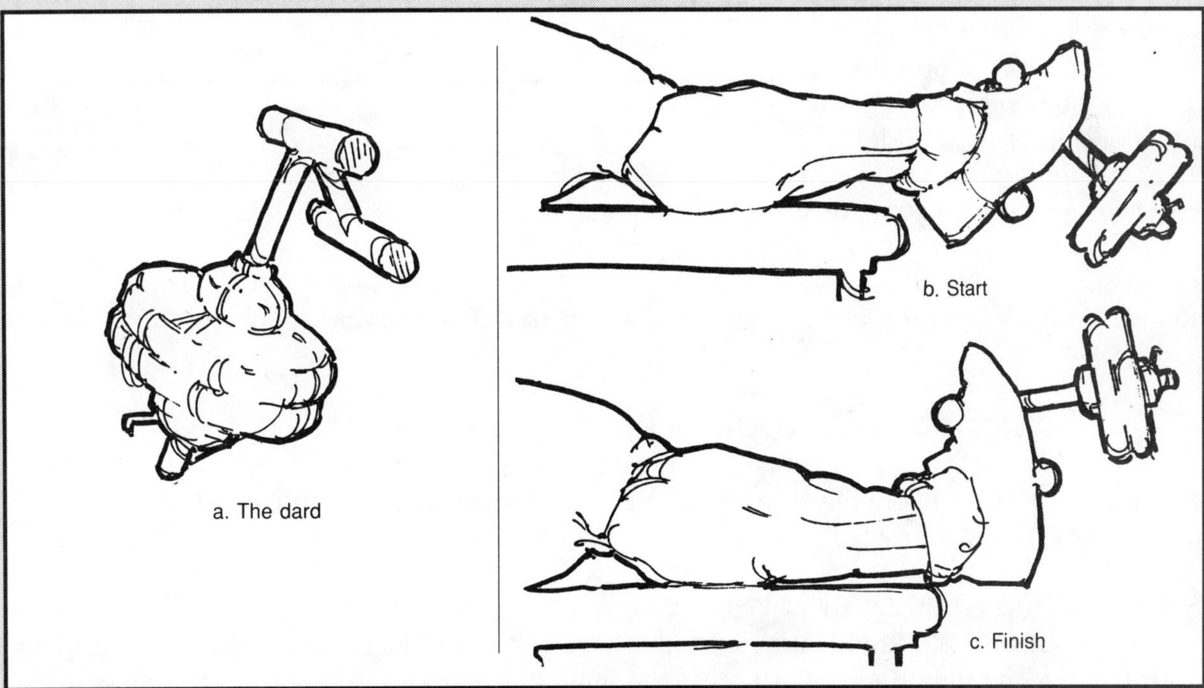

Fig. 25

† Dards are available from Health For Life, 8033 Sunset Blvd. Suite 483, Los Angeles CA 90046 (800) 874-5339 or (800) 623-9983 (in Calif.).

Using the Iron Boot

The *iron boot* is your second-best choice. Unlike the *dard*, the iron boot requires you to work each leg separately. This not only increases workout time but also calls for greater focus and care, given the combined effect of (1) the amount of weight necessary to properly stress the dorsiflexors, and (2) the relative instability of a one- versus two-leg exercise.

Prepare by screwing the bar supplied with the boot into the socket on the boot's toe. Strap the boot to the bottom of your left shoe. Make sure the straps are pulled *tight*. Place a small amount of weight on the bar and tighten the retaining clamp.

Sit on the edge of a tall stool or table with your legs dangling (Fig. 26-a). Slowly bend your ankle so the front of your foot moves up as far as possible toward your shin (Fig. 26-b). Don't let your foot pronate or supinate (shift to either side).

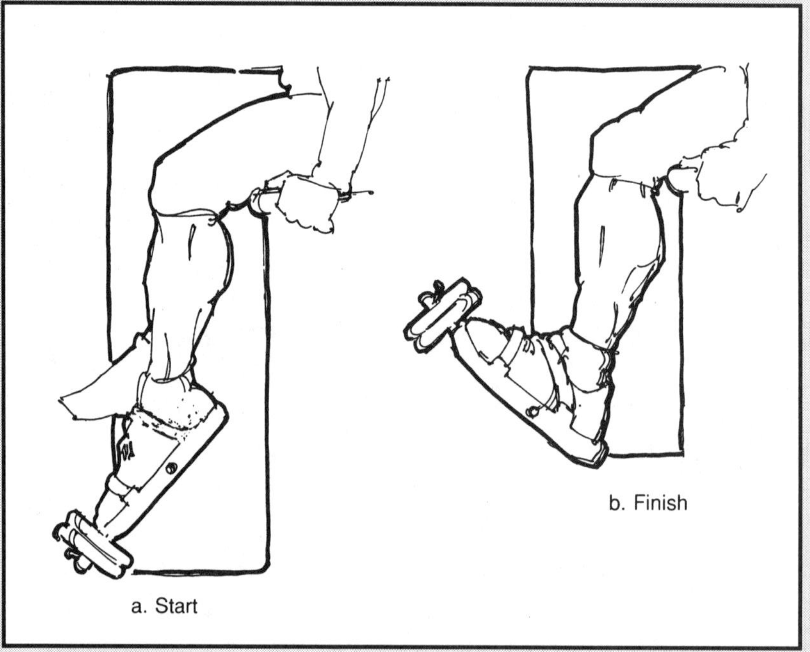

Fig. 26

Hold for a second at peak, then lower your foot back to the starting position, feeling for the stretch in the anterior tibialis.

Repeat for each foot for the number of reps specified in the program section.

Using a Rubber Strap

A *rubber strap* is probably the simplest and least expensive device you can use for performing this exercise. Either a big rubber band or a loop of surgical tubing will do.†

Set yourself up as illustrated in Figure 27-a below. Of course you don't have to use this exact arrangement. Workout benches or other furniture could be substituted for the chairs in the drawing. The important point is that the line of resistance imposed by the rubber strap be the same as that indicated by the arrow in the illustration.

† You can buy surgical tubing for a dollar or two at any medical supply house.

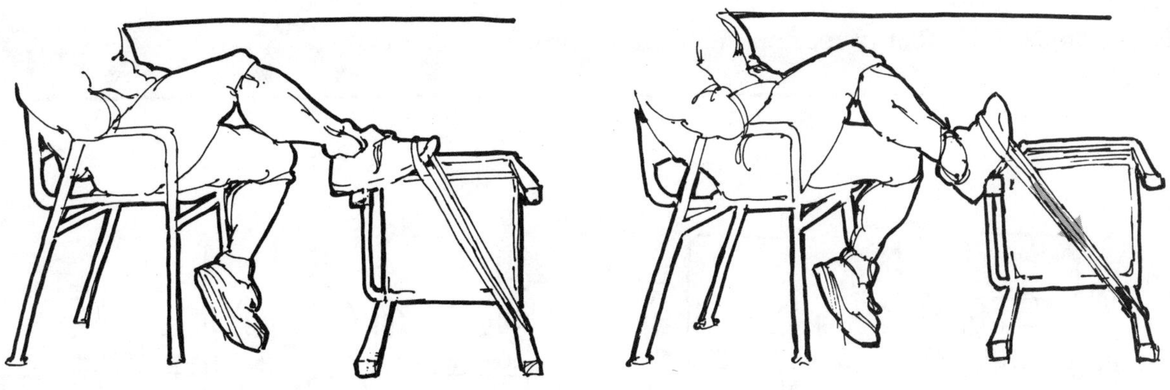

Fig. 27

Bend your ankle so the front of your foot moves up as far as possible toward your shin (Fig. 27-b). Don't let your foot pronate or supinate (shift to either side).

Hold for a second at peak, then slowly relax, feeling for the stretch in the anterior tibialis.

Repeat for each foot for the number of reps specified in the program section.

FOOT INWARD ROCKS

prime mover: supinators

This exercise works the ankle supination muscles. Strengthening these muscles—and balancing their strength with that of their opposing group, the pronators—is essential for maximizing footwork speed and ankle stability.

The exercise can be performed using different equipment. Best choice: rubber strap. The Iron Boot is adequate but not ideal.†

Using a Rubber Strap

Set up as illustrated in Figure 28-a below. Once again, this is only an example of the appropriate arrangement. The important point is that the lines of resistance imposed by the rubber straps be the same as those indicated by the arrows in the illustration.

† One measure of an exercise's efficiency is the accuracy with which it imposes resistance against the line of force generated by the target muscle group. For performing Foot Inward Rocks, the rubber strap does a better job of this than the Iron Boot. See our text, *Secrets of Advanced Bodybuilders,* for a complete explanation of lines of force and resistance.

Rock your feet inward as far as possible (Fig. 28-b). Hold for a second at peak, then return to the starting position.

Repeat for the number of reps specified in the program section.

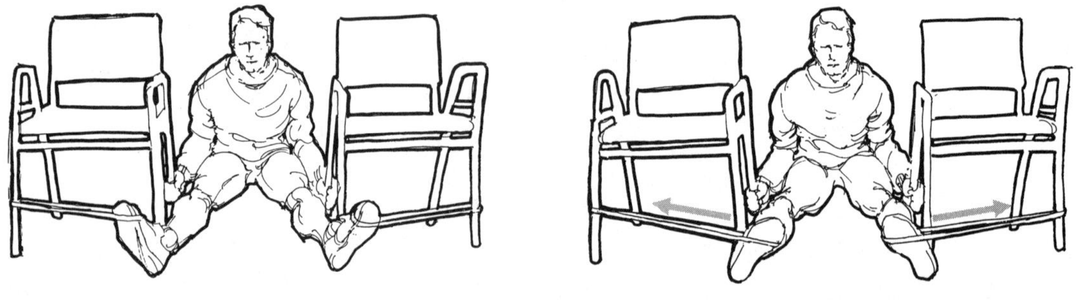

a. Start b. Finish

Fig. 28

Using the Iron Boot

Screw the bar supplied with the Iron Boot into the socket on the inside edge of the boot. Strap the boot to the bottom of your right shoe. Make sure the straps are pulled *tight*. Place a small amount of weight on the bar and tighten the retaining clamp.

Sit on the edge of a tall stool or table with your legs dangling (Fig. 29-a). Slowly rock your foot inward, as indicated in Figure 29-b.

Hold for a second at peak, then lower your foot back to the starting position.

Repeat for each foot for the number of reps specified in the program section.

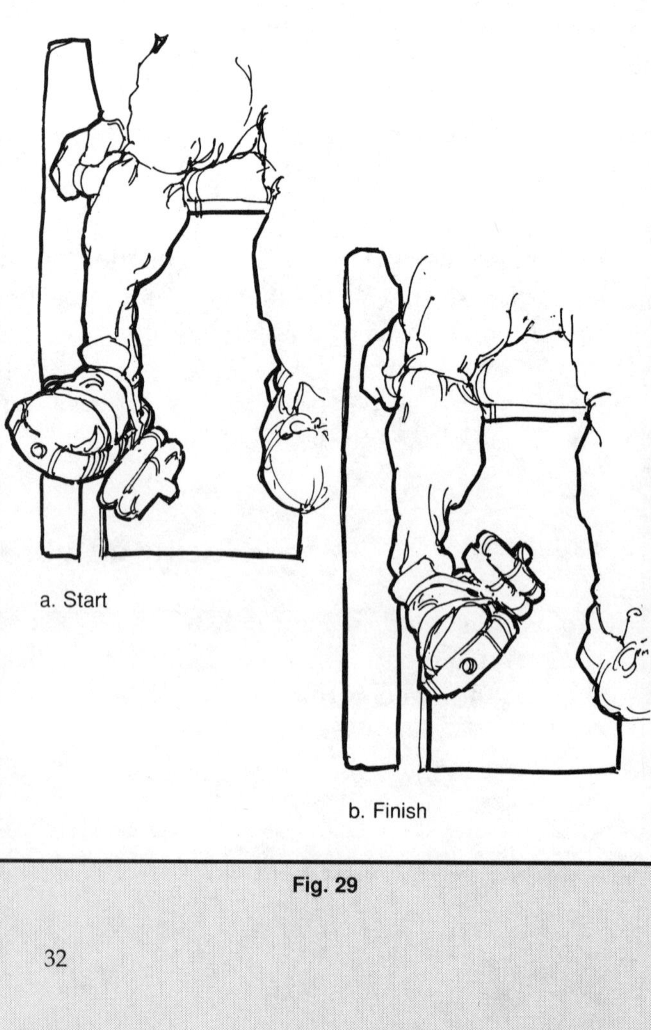

a. Start b. Finish

Fig. 29

FOOT OUTWARD ROCKS

prime mover: pronators

This exercise works the ankle pronation muscles. Strengthening these muscles—and balancing their strength with that of their opposing group, the supinators (worked by the previous exercise)—is essential for maximizing footwork speed and ankle stability.

Again, the exercise can be performed using different equipment. Again, best choice: rubber strap. The Iron Boot is adequate but not ideal (see footnote from Foot Inward Rocks).

Using a Rubber Strap

Set up as illustrated in Figure 30-a below. Once again, if you use another arrangement, make sure the lines of resistance imposed by the rubber straps are the same as those indicated by the arrows in the illustration.

Rock your feet outward as far as possible (Fig. 30-b). Hold for a second at peak, then return to the starting position.

Repeat for the number of reps specified in the program section.

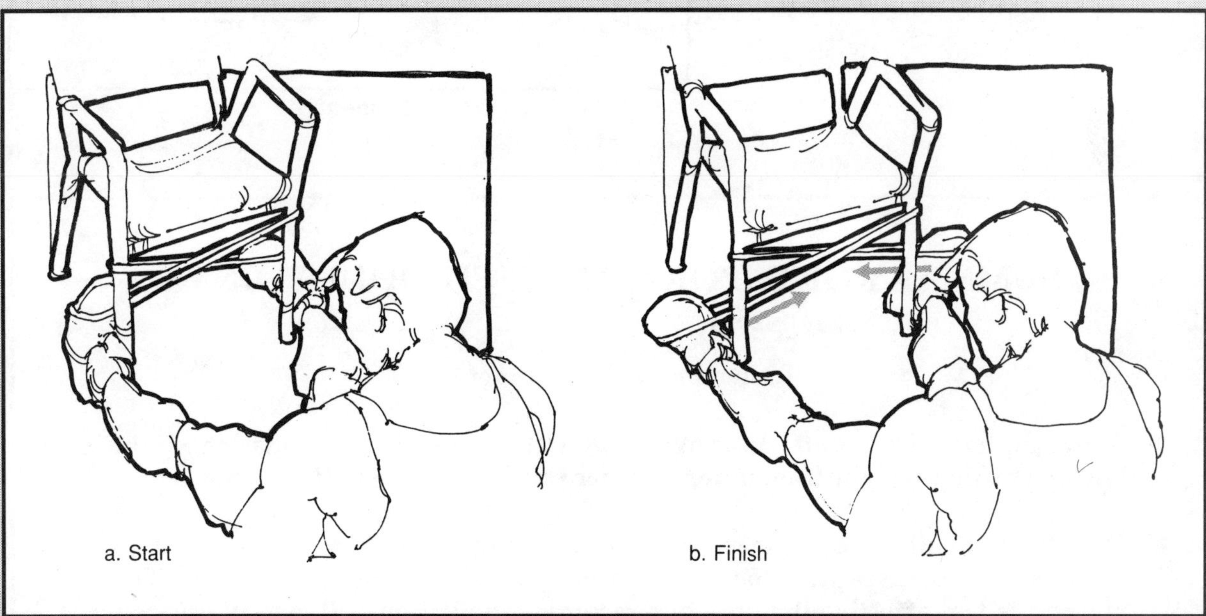

Fig. 30

Using the Iron Boot

Screw the bar supplied with the Iron Boot into the socket on the outside edge of the boot. Strap the boot to the bottom of your right shoe. Make sure the straps are pulled *tight*. Place a small amount of weight on the bar and tighten the retaining clamp.

Sit on the edge of a tall stool or table with your legs dangling (Fig. 31-a). Slowly rock your foot outward, as indicated in Figure 31-b.

Hold for a second at peak, then lower your foot back to the starting position.

Repeat for each foot for the number of reps specified in the program section.

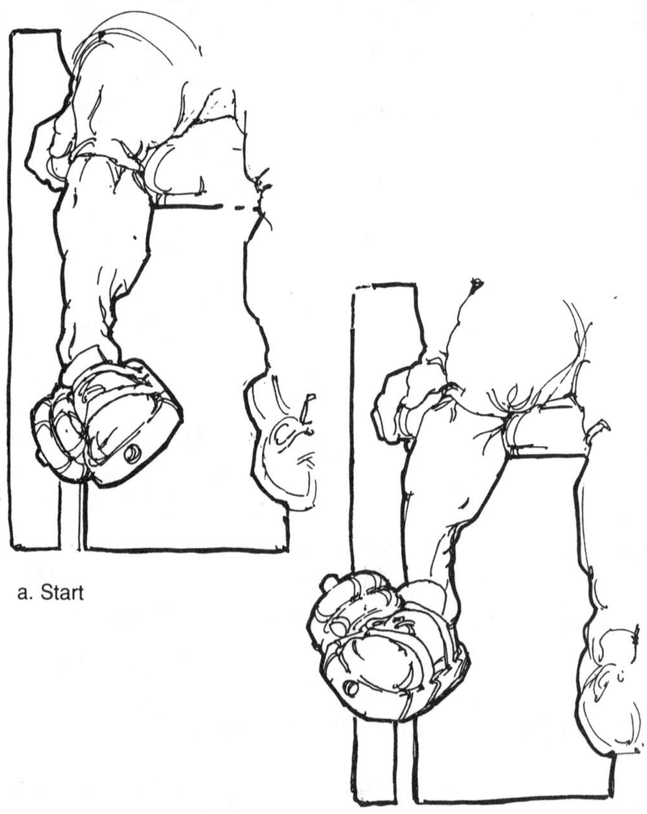

a. Start

b. Finish

Fig. 31

SUMMARY OF IMPORTANT TECHNIQUE POINTS

To maximize development...

- **Shift emphasis from outer to inner plantar flexor heads by pronating slightly—by shifting weight from outer to inner portions of the balls of your feet.**
- ***Do not* shift calf raise emphasis from outer to inner plantar flexor heads by doing some exercises with toes pointed out, some with toes pointed in. This method is less effective than the one recommended above. It also places considerably more stress on the ankle and knee joints, increasing risk of injury.**
- **Perform the first part of each calf raise set with legs straight (to stress both soleus and gastroc), then perform the second part with knees bent (to stress primarily the soleus).**

FLEXIBILITY

Any muscle that undergoes repeated contraction *and is not repeatedly stretched* will eventually shorten—it will lose flexibility.

The calves are no exception. In fact, since they contract with every step you take (not to mention with every athletic endeavor involving a push-off), they often end up tight enough to seriously increase your risk of injury. A common result: Achilles tendonitis, inflammation of the large tendon that runs down the back of your lower calf and connects to the top of your heel bone. Many, many athletes (especially runners) needlessly suffer from this condition simply because they don't maintain sufficient flexibility in their plantar flexors.

The exercises in this section are designed to ensure you develop—and maintain—calf flexibility. They only take a minute or two. And performing them along with the **Maximum Calves** routines is *synergistic*: Research shows that, if you do flexibility work after resistance training, you develop more flexibility more quickly, experience much less of the pain usually associated with stretching, and suffer less soreness from the weight workout!

SINGLE-LEG CALF STRETCH

target: plantar flexors

Presented below are three ways to perform this stretch, varying in intensity from mild to severe. You will have to experiment to determine which version is best for you.

Mild Version — Standing

Stand about four feet away from a wall. Step forward with your right foot, keeping your left foot in place. Support yourself against the wall with right knee bent, left leg straight, *left heel flat against the floor* (Fig. 32-a).

Lean in toward the wall, keeping your left leg straight and left heel against the floor (Fig. 32-b). Feel for the stretch in your plantar flexors. Relax into the stretch, playing the edges of your flexibility for about 15 seconds.

Repeat with your left leg forward.

If the stretch is too easy, position your left foot farther from the wall (Fig. 32-c); if too difficult, move your left foot in toward the wall.

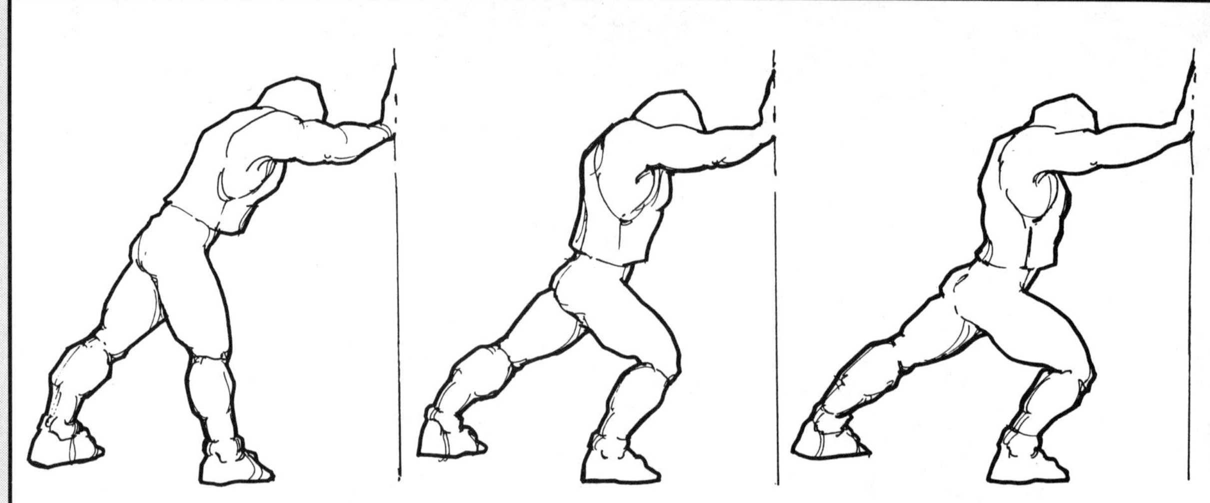

a. Start b. Relax into stretch c. Harder—rear foot farther back

Fig. 32

Moderate Version — Crouching

Get into "sprinting position" as illustrated in Figure 33-a. Your rear leg should be straight, your rear heel *off the ground.*

Rock your weight back onto your rear leg, feeling for the stretch in your plantar flexors (Fig. 33-b). Make sure you keep the rear leg straight. Relax into the stretch for about fifteen seconds. Don't bounce. Repeat with your other leg back.

If the stretch is too easy, increase the distance from hands to rear foot, and drop your hips down lower while performing the stretch (Fig. 33-c). If it's too hard, do the reverse—decrease the distance from your hands to your rear foot, and keep your hips up higher.

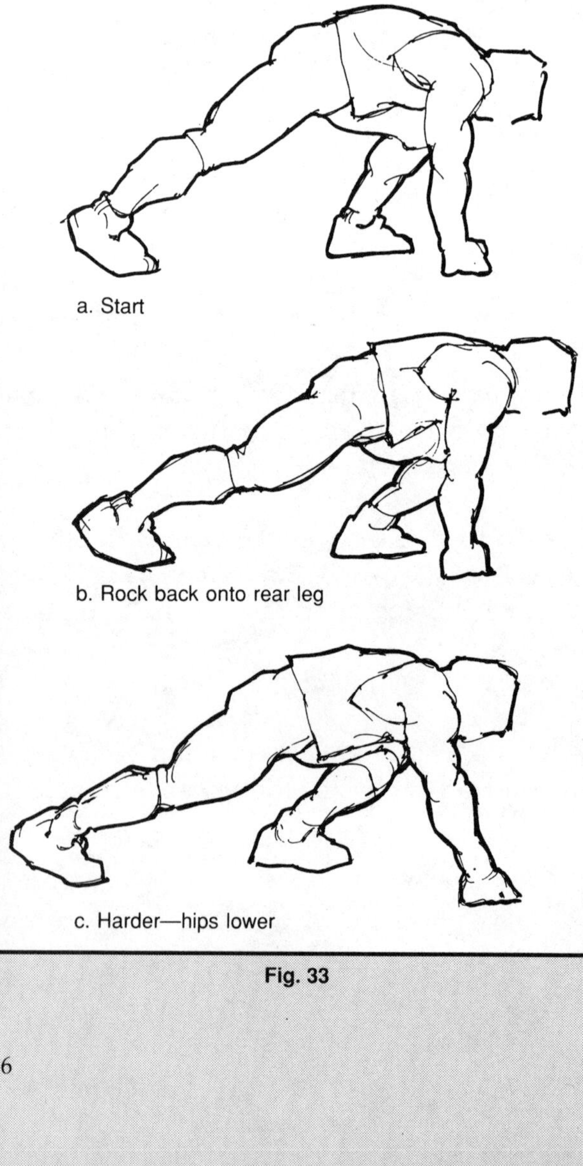

a. Start

b. Rock back onto rear leg

c. Harder—hips lower

Fig. 33

Severe Version — Using a Block

Place the ball of your right foot against the edge of a low block—five to six inches high is perfect. Lean forward, supporting yourself on a stool or bench, keeping your right leg straight. Try to touch your right heel to the ground (Fig. 34-a). Relax into the stretch for about fifteen seconds, playing your edges. Repeat with left foot against the block.

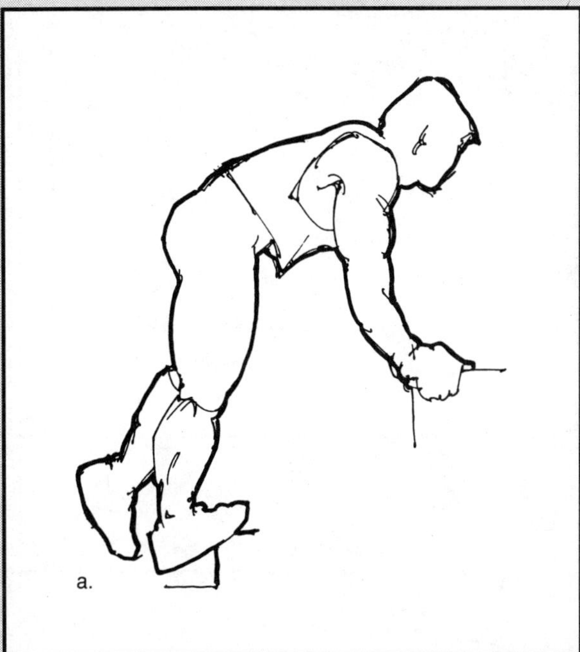

a.

You can increase the intensity several ways. From least to most severe:

- Lean farther forward (Fig. 34-b);
- Place the heel of your left foot against the toes of your right and push back gently (Fig. 34-c);
- Extend your left leg back and up as you perform the stretch (Fig. 34-d).

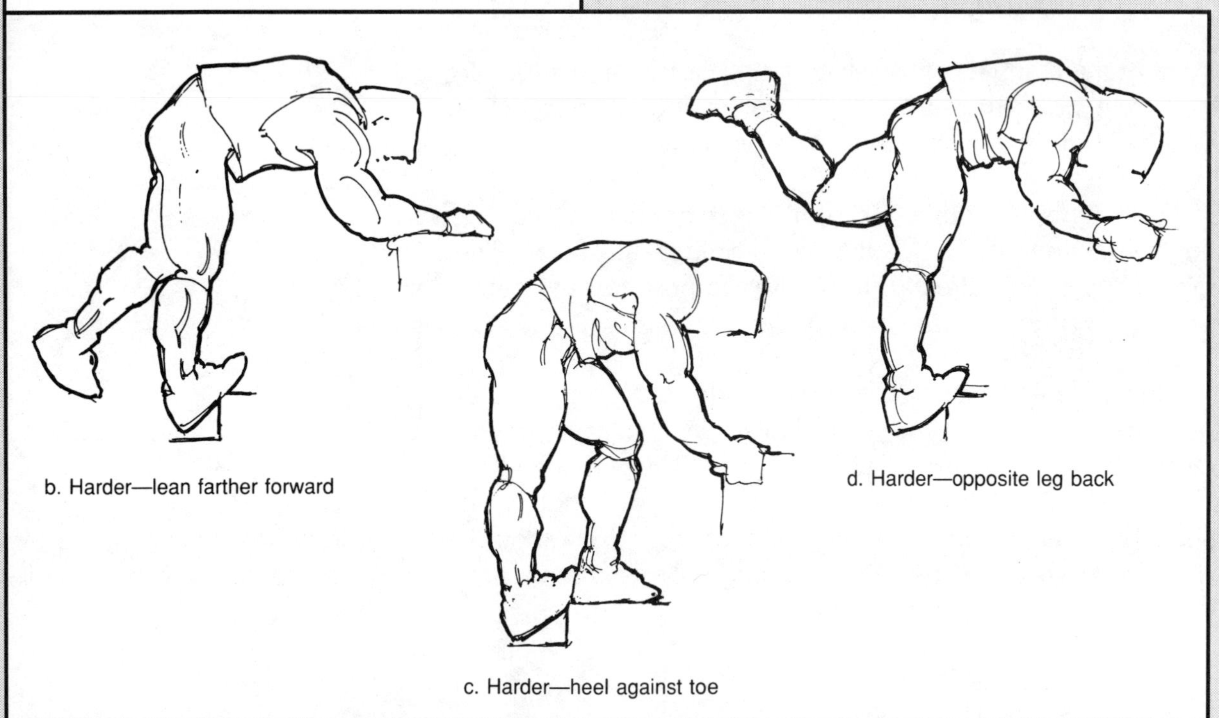

b. Harder—lean farther forward

c. Harder—heel against toe

d. Harder—opposite leg back

Fig. 34

TOES POINTED STRETCH

target: dorsiflexors

Take your shoes off and sit down on the ground. Place your right hand against the back of your right heel, right thumb in the middle of the sole of your right foot. Place your left thumb on the sole next to your right thumb, and curl the fingers of your left hand around the inside of your right foot, so they lie on the tops of your toes (Fig. 35).

Gently plantar flex your foot by bending your toes down with your left hand while pushing forward on your heel with your right. Feel for the stretch in the anterior tibialis. Hold for 5-10 seconds, then release.

Repeat for your left foot.

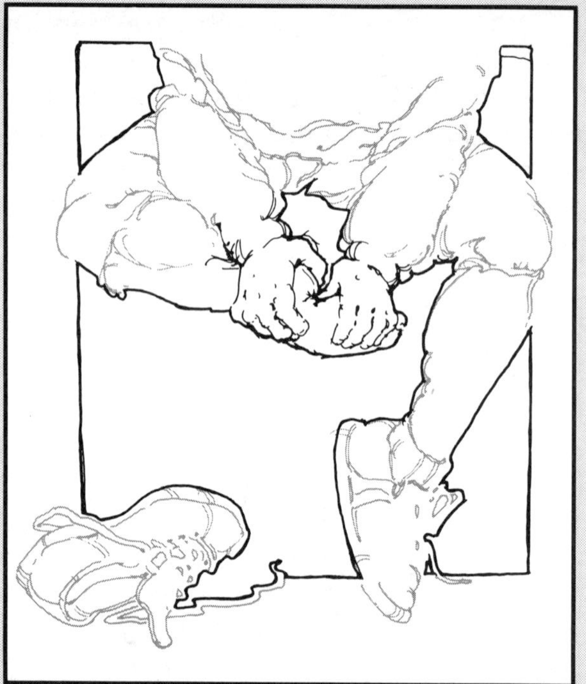

Fig. 35

ANKLE ROCKED-IN CALF STRETCH

target: pronators and plantar flexors

This is an advanced stretch that requires considerable *hamstring* flexibility just to get into position. It stretches the hamstrings as well as the ankle pronators.

Sit on a table with your right leg extended along the edge and your left leg acting as a balance support. The table should be tall enough to allow almost full extension of your supporting leg.

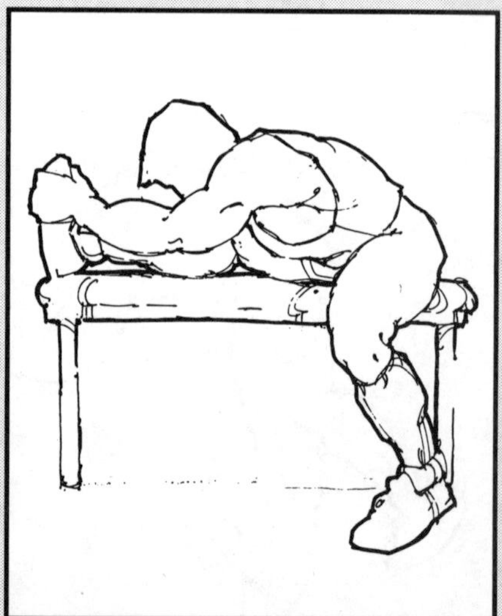

Fig. 36

Bring your left hand across your body and grab the ball of your right foot; bend your knee slightly, even if you don't have to. Make sure your foot is supinated (rolled inward) (Fig. 36). Pull back on the ball of your foot while simultaneously trying to straighten your leg. You should feel the stretch primarily along the outside of your calf but also to some extent in your hamstrings. Hold for fifteen seconds, then release.

Repeat for your left leg.

THE ROUTINES

Both sets of routines detailed in this section will increase overall calf strength. Beyond that, the first targets the needs of the bodybuilder—use it to *pile on the MASS*! The second targets the needs of the martial artist or other athlete whose success depends on fast footwork—use it to *increase footwork speed and ankle stability.*

Whichever routine you use, take it easy at first! Work your way up through the levels, changing only when your progress slows or your workout begins to feel too easy. The idea is to find a balance between getting all you can out of a level, and consistently providing sufficient overload to stimulate growth. Keep in mind, though—if you move up too soon, all you're doing is forcing yourself to work harder and longer than necessary to achieve the results you want.

MASS AND STRENGTH ROUTINE

Intended for: bodybuilders, others interested in increasing calf mass and strength

This routine concentrates on the plantar flexors, but stimulates their opposing group, the dorsiflexors—as well as the other major muscle group pair in the calves, the supinators and pronators—enough to ensure balanced calf development and improved functional strength.

To reap maximum benefit from the routine, you must do your part to maintain a high Fatigue/Tension level by adhering strictly to the rest times indicated. That, in many cases, means *no rest at all!*

LEVEL A — Mass and Strength

Warmup

1 set	Standing Toe Pull-Backs	*1 minute*
1 set	Calf Bounces	*1 minute*

Exercises

2 sets No rest between sets	Single-Leg Calf Raises	*Each set:* *Leg straight* *6-8 reps, outer head* *4-6 reps, inner head* *Leg bent* *6-8 reps, outer head* *4-6 reps, inner head* *Repeat for other leg*

— no rest —

1 set	Seated Toe Pull-Backs	*8-10 reps*

Stretches

1 set 1 set 1 set	Single-Leg Calf Stretch .... *5 to 10 seconds each leg* Toes Pointed Stretch .... *5 to 10 seconds each leg* Ankle Rocked-In Calf Stretch .... *5 to 10 seconds each leg*

LEVEL B — Mass and Strength

Warmup

1 set 1 set	Standing Toe Pull-Backs .... *1 minute* Calf Bounces .... *1 minute*

Exercises

3 sets No rest between sets	Single-Leg Calf Raises .... *Each set:* *Leg straight* *6-8 reps, outer head* *4-6 reps, inner head* *Leg bent* *6-8 reps, outer head* *4-6 reps, inner head* *Repeat for other leg*

— no rest —

1 set	Seated Toe Pull-Backs .... *8-10 reps*

— no rest —

1 set	Foot Inward Rocks .... *8-10 reps*

— no rest —

1 set	Foot Outward Rocks .... *8-10 reps*

Stretches

1 set 1 set 1 set	Single-Leg Calf Stretch .... *5 to 10 seconds each leg* Toes Pointed Stretch .... *5 to 10 seconds each leg* Ankle Rocked-In Calf Stretch .... *5 to 10 seconds each leg*

Warmup

1 set	Standing Toe Pull-Backs .... *1 minute*
1 set	Calf Bounces .... *1 minute*

Exercises

3 sets No rest between sets	Single-Leg Calf Raises .... *Each set:* *Leg straight* *6-8 reps, outer head* *4-6 reps, inner head* *Leg bent* *6-8 reps, outer head* *4-6 reps, inner head* *Repeat for other leg*
	— no rest —
2 compound sets No rest between sets	Donkey or Nautilus Calf Raises .... *Each set:* *Legs straight* *6-8 reps, outer head* *4-6 reps, inner head* *Legs bent* *6-8 reps, outer head* *4-6 reps, inner head* Calf Rock-Ups .... *20 seconds*
	— no rest —
1 set	Seated Toe Pull-Backs .... *8-10 reps*
	— no rest —
1 set	Foot Inward Rocks .... *8-10 reps*
	— no rest —
1 set	Foot Outward Rocks .... *8-10 reps*

Stretches

1 set	Single-Leg Calf Stretch .... *5 to 10 seconds each leg*
1 set	Toes Pointed Stretch .... *5 to 10 seconds each leg*
1 set	Ankle Rocked-In Calf Stretch .... *5 to 10 seconds each leg*

Warmup

1 set	Standing Toe Pull-Backs..*1 minute*
1 set	Calf Bounces..*1 minute*

Exercises

3 sets No rest between sets	Single-Leg Calf Raises ....*Each set:* *Leg straight* *6-8 reps, outer head* *4-6 reps, inner head* *Leg bent* *6-8 reps, outer head* *4-6 reps, inner head* *Repeat for other leg*

— no rest —

3 compound sets No rest between sets	Donkey or Nautilus Calf Raises..........................*Each set:* *Legs straight* *6-8 reps, outer head* *4-6 reps, inner head* *Legs bent* *6-8 reps, outer head* *4-6 reps, inner head* Calf Rock-Ups ....*20 seconds*

— no rest —

1 set	Standing Calf Raises ....*Each set:* *Legs straight* *6-8 reps, outer head* *4-6 reps, inner head* *Legs bent* *6-8 reps, outer head* *4-6 reps, inner head*

— no rest —

1 set	Seated Calf Raises ....*6-8 reps, outer head* *4-6 reps, inner head*

— no rest —

1 set	Seated Toe Pull-Backs..*8-10 reps*

— no rest —

1 set	Foot Inward Rocks..*8-10 reps*

— no rest —

1 set	Foot Outward Rocks..*8-10 reps*

Stretches

1 set	Single-Leg Calf Stretch...*5 to 10 seconds each leg*
1 set	Toes Pointed Stretch...*5 to 10 seconds each leg*
1 set	Ankle Rocked-In Calf Stretch...............................*5 to 10 seconds each leg*

Warmup

1 set	Standing Toe Pull-Backs..*1 minute*
1 set	Calf Bounces...*1 minute*

Exercises

2 sets No rest between sets	Single-Leg Calf Raises ....*Each set:* *Leg straight* *6-8 reps, outer head* *4-6 reps, inner head* *Leg bent* *6-8 reps, outer head* *4-6 reps, inner head* *Repeat for other leg*

— no rest —

3 compound sets No rest between sets	Donkey or Nautilus Calf Raises...........................*Each set:* *Legs straight* *6-8 reps, outer head* *4-6 reps, inner head* *Legs bent* *6-8 reps, outer head* *4-6 reps, inner head* Calf Rock-Ups ....*20 seconds*

— no rest —

1 compound set	Standing Calf Raises, ***outer*** head.........................*Each set:* *Legs straight* *6-8 reps* *Legs bent* *4-6 reps* Calf Rock-Ups...*20 seconds*

— no rest —

1 compound set	Standing Calf Raises, ***inner*** head ....*Each set:* *Legs straight* *6-8 reps* *Legs bent* *4-6 reps* Calf Rock-Ups ....*20 seconds*

— no rest —

1 set	Seated Calf Raises, ***outer*** head............................*8-10 reps*

— 10 seconds rest —

1 set	Seated Calf Raises, ***inner*** head............................*8-10 reps*

— no rest —

2 sets 10 seconds rest between sets	Seated Toe Pull-Backs ....*8-10 reps*

— no rest —

2 sets	Foot Inward Rocks..*8-10 reps*

— no rest —

2 sets	Foot Outward Rocks..*8-10 reps*

Stretches

1 set	Single-Leg Calf Stretch..*5 to 10 seconds each leg*
1 set	Toes Pointed Stretch..*5 to 10 seconds each leg*
1 set	Ankle Rocked-In Calf Stretch...............................*5 to 10 seconds each leg*

FOOTWORK SPEED/ANKLE STABILITY ROUTINE

Intended for: martial artists, others interested in increasing footwork speed and ankle stability.

Compared to the MASS routine, this routine contains less work for the plantar flexors and considerably more for the pronators and supinators.

LEVEL A — Speed, Stability, and Strength

Warmup

1 set	Standing Toe Pull-Backs..*1 minute*
1 set	Calf Bounces..*1 minute*

Exercises

1 set	Single-Leg Calf Raises ....*Each set:* *Leg straight* *6-8 reps, outer head* *4-6 reps, inner head* *Leg bent* *6-8 reps, outer head* *4-6 reps, inner head* *Repeat for other leg*

— no rest —

1 set	Seated Toe Pull-Backs..*8-10 reps*

— no rest —

1 set	Foot Inward Rocks ....*8-10 reps*

— no rest —

1 set	Foot Outward Rocks...*8-10 reps*

Stretches

1 set	Single-Leg Calf Stretch ....*5 to 10 seconds each leg*
1 set	Toes Pointed Stretch ....*5 to 10 seconds each leg*
1 set	Ankle Rocked-In Calf Stretch...............................*5 to 10 seconds each leg*

Warmup

1 set	Standing Toe Pull-Backs	*1 minute*
1 set	Calf Bounces	*1 minute*

Exercises

2 sets No rest between sets	Single-Leg Calf Raises	*Each set:* *Leg straight* *6-8 reps, outer head* *4-6 reps, inner head* *Leg bent* *6-8 reps, outer head* *4-6 reps, inner head* *Repeat for other leg*
	— no rest —	
1 compound set	Donkey or Nautilus Calf Raises	*Each set:* *Legs straight* *6-8 reps, outer head* *4-6 reps, inner head* *Legs bent* *6-8 reps, outer head* *4-6 reps, inner head*
	Calf Rock-Ups	*20 seconds*
	— no rest —	
2 sets	Seated Toe Pull-Backs	*8-10 reps*
	— no rest —	
2 sets	Foot Inward Rocks	*8-10 reps*
	— no rest —	
2 sets	Foot Outward Rocks	*8-10 reps*

Stretches

1 set	Single-Leg Calf Stretch	*5 to 10 seconds each leg*
1 set	Toes Pointed Stretch	*5 to 10 seconds each leg*
1 set	Ankle Rocked-In Calf Stretch	*5 to 10 seconds each leg*

Warmup

1 set	Standing Toe Pull-Backs......*1 minute*
1 set	Calf Bounces......*1 minute*

Exercises

2 sets No rest between sets	Single-Leg Calf Raises......*Each set:* *Leg straight* *6-8 reps, outer head* *4-6 reps, inner head* *Leg bent* *6-8 reps, outer head* *4-6 reps, inner head* *Repeat for other leg*

— no rest —

2 compound sets No rest between sets	Donkey or Nautilus Calf Raises......*Each set:* *Legs straight* *6-8 reps, outer head* *4-6 reps, inner head* *Legs bent* *6-8 reps, outer head* *4-6 reps, inner head* Calf Rock-Ups......*20 seconds*

— no rest —

3 sets 10 seconds rest between sets	Seated Toe Pull-Backs......*8-10 reps*

— no rest —

3 sets 10 seconds rest between sets	Foot Inward Rocks......*8-10 reps*

— no rest —

3 sets 10 seconds rest between sets	Foot Outward Rocks..........*8-10 reps*

Stretches

1 set	Single-Leg Calf Stretch..........*5 to 10 seconds each leg*
1 set	Toes Pointed Stretch..........*5 to 10 seconds each leg*
1 set	Ankle Rocked-In Calf Stretch..........*5 to 10 seconds each leg*

LEVEL A

Single Leg C.R.

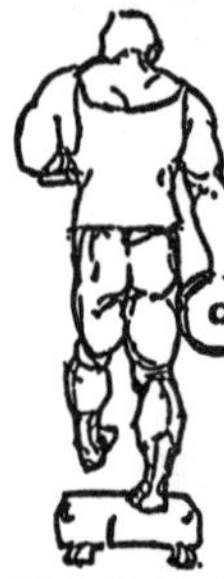

LS0: 6-8 reps
LSI: 4-6 reps
LBO: 6-8 reps
LBI: 4-6 reps

2 Sets

Seated Toe Pull-Backs

8-10 reps

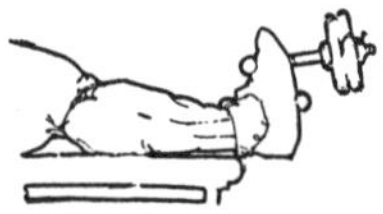

1 Set

LEVEL B

Single Leg C.R.

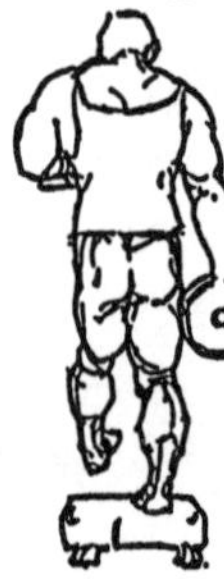

LS0: 6-8 reps
LSI: 4-6 reps
LBO: 6-8 reps
LBI: 4-6 reps

3 Sets

Seated Toe Pull-Backs

8-10 reps

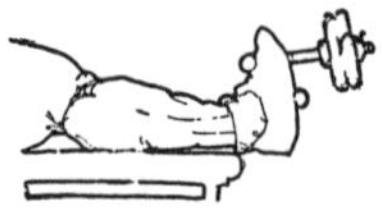

1 Set

Foot Inward Rocks

8-10 reps

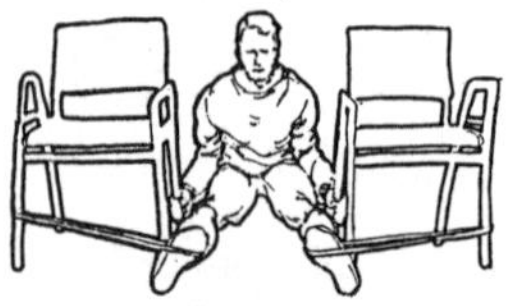

1 Set

Foot Outward Rocks

8-10 reps

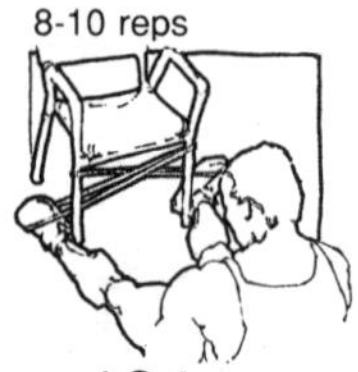

1 Set

LEVEL 1

Single Leg C.R.

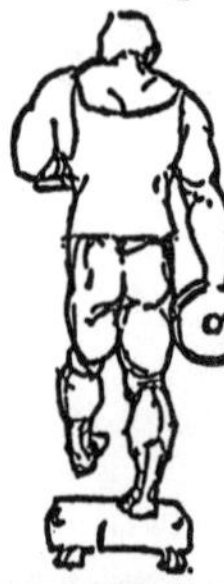

LS0: 6-8 reps
LSI: 4-6 reps
LBO: 6-8 reps
LBI: 4-6 reps

2 Sets

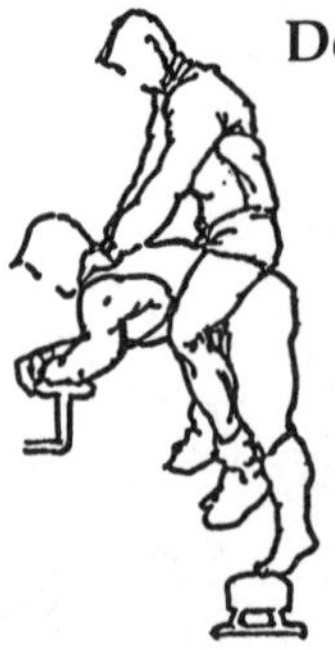

Donkey C.R.

LS0: 6-8 reps
LSI: 4-6 reps
LBO: 6-8 reps
LBI: 4-6 reps

Calf Rock-ups

20 secs.

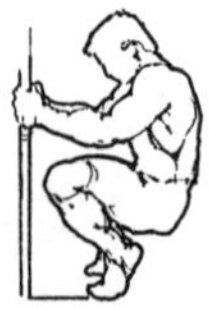

2 Compound Sets

Seated Toe Pull-Backs

8-10 reps

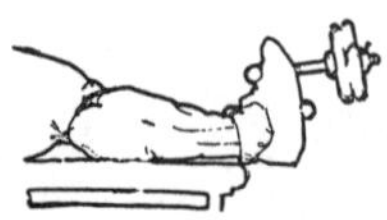

1 Set

LEVEL 2

Single Leg C.R.

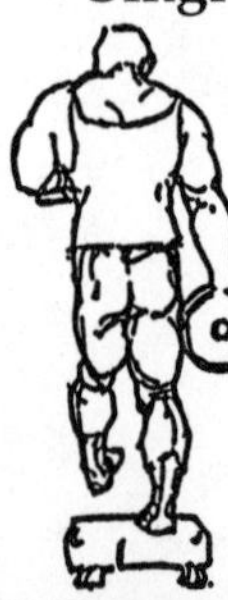

LS0: 6-8 reps
LSI: 4-6 reps
LBO: 6-8 reps
LBI: 4-6 reps

3 Sets

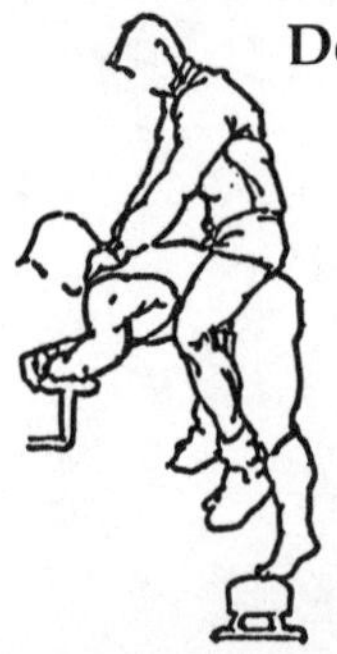

Donkey C.R.

LS0: 6-8 reps
LSI: 4-6 reps
LBO: 6-8 reps
LBI: 4-6 reps

Calf Rock-ups

20 secs.

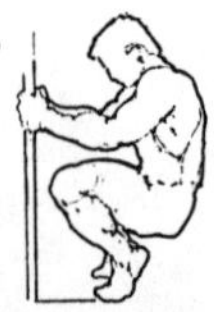

3 Compound Sets

Standing C.R.

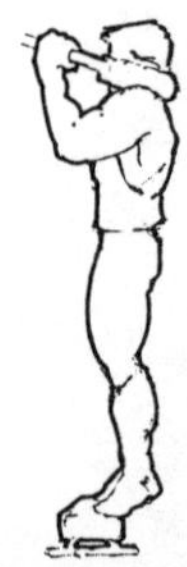

LS0: 6-8 reps
LSI: 4-6 reps
LBO: 6-8 reps
LBI: 4-6 reps

1 Set

LEVEL 3

Single Leg C.R.

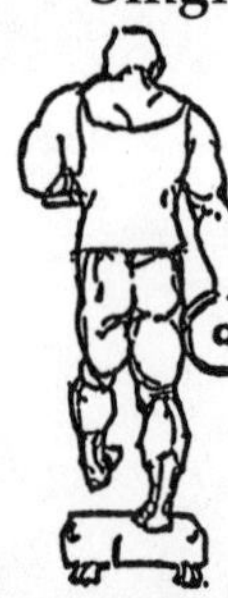

LS0: 6-8 reps
LSI: 4-6 reps
LBO: 6-8 reps
LBI: 4-6 reps

2 Sets

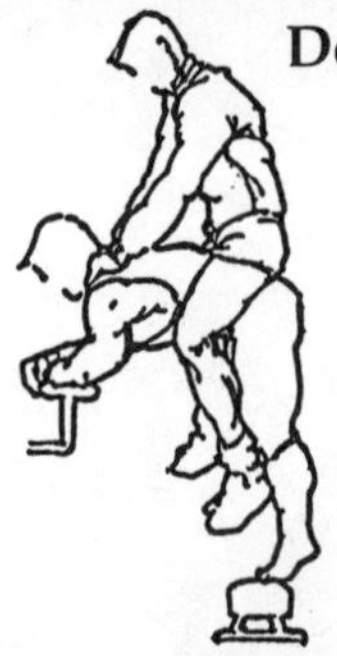

Donkey C.R.

LS0: 6-8 reps
LSI: 4-6 reps
LBO: 6-8 reps
LBI: 4-6 reps

Calf Rock-ups

20 secs.

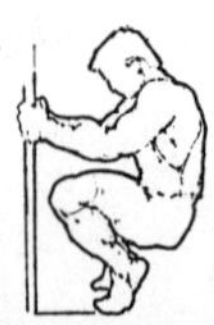

3 Compound Sets

Standing C.R.

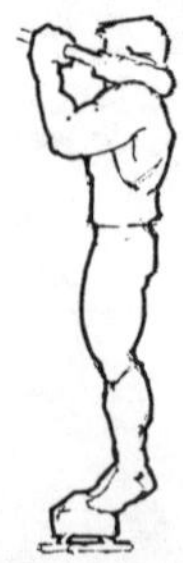

LS0: 6-8 reps
LBO: 6-8 reps

Calf Rock-ups

20 secs.

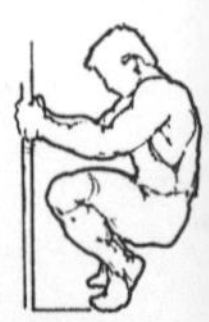

1 Compound Set

Mass and Strength Routines *Illustrated*

KEY

LSO = Legs straight, outer calf
LSI = Legs straight, inner calf
LBO = Legs bent, outer calf
LBI = Legs bent, inner calf

Begin all levels with the **Warmup** routine illustrated on the bottom of page 52.

End all levels with the **Stretch** routine illustrated on the bottom of page 53.

Foot Inward Rocks

8-10 reps

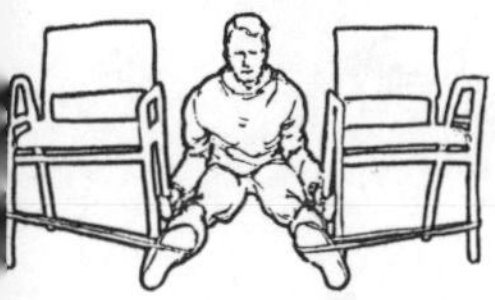

1 Set

Foot Outward Rocks

8-10 reps

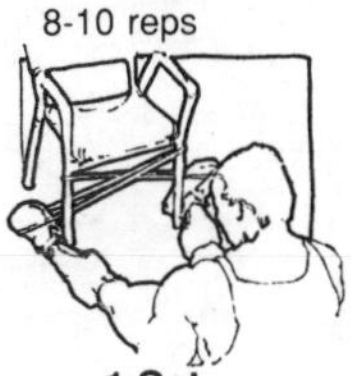

1 Set

Seated C.R.

O: 6-8 reps
I: 4-6 reps

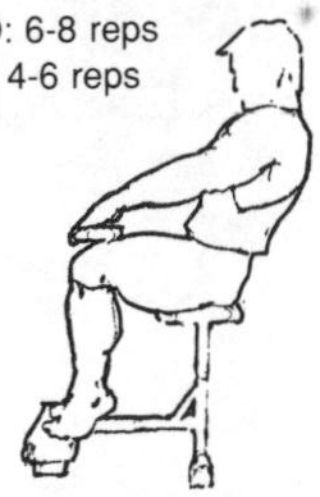

1 Set

Seated Toe Pull-Backs

8-10 reps

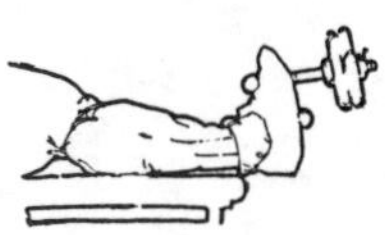

1 Set

Foot Inward Rocks

8-10 reps

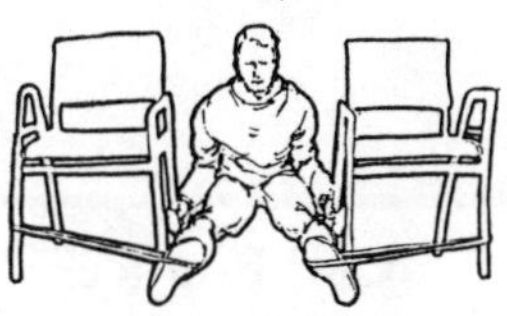

1 Set

Foot Outward Rocks

8-10 reps

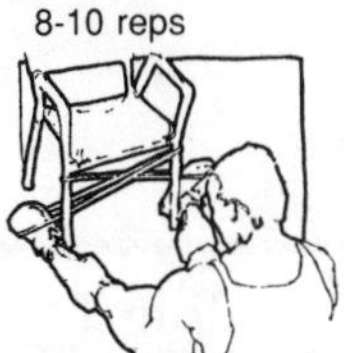

1 Set

Standing C.R.

LSI: 6-8 reps
LBI: 6-8 reps

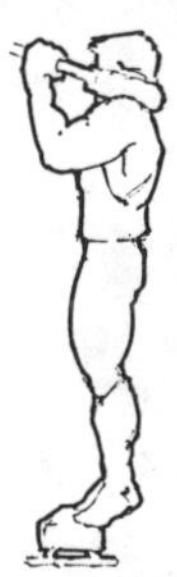

Calf Rock-ups

20 secs.

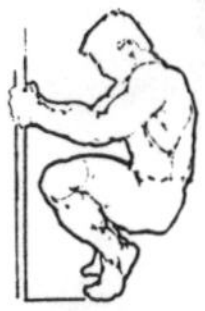

1 Compound Set

Seated C.R.

8-10 reps

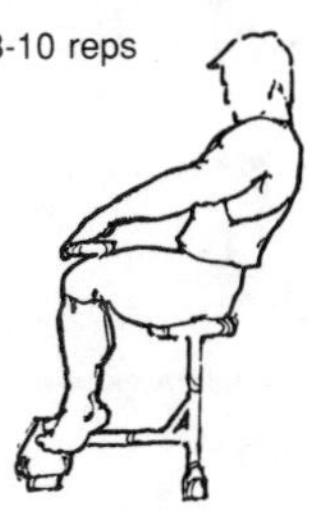

1 Outer, 1 Inner

Seated Toe Pull-Backs

8-10 reps

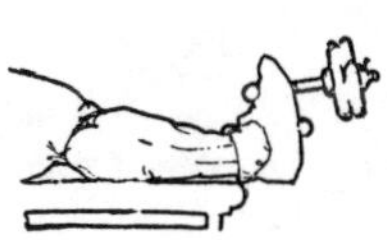

2 Sets

Foot Inward Rocks

8-10 reps

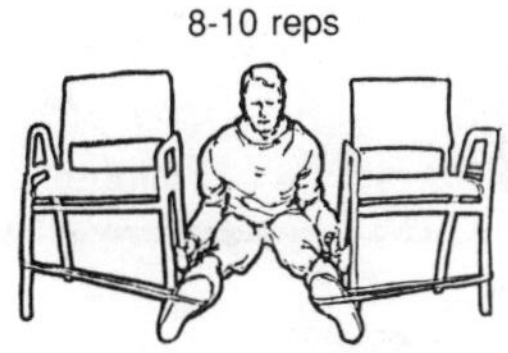

2 Sets

Foot Outward Rocks

8-10 reps

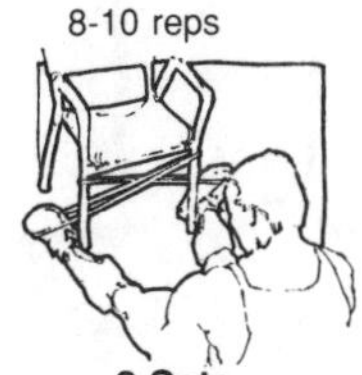

2 Sets

LEVEL A

Single Leg C.R.

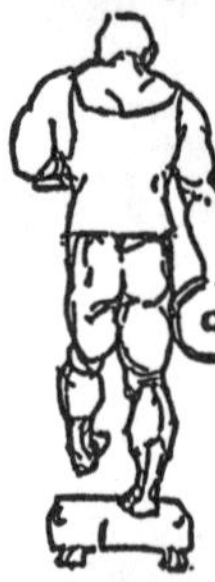

LS0: 6-8 reps
LSI: 4-6 reps
LBO: 6-8 reps
LBI: 4-6 reps

1 Set

Seated Toe Pull-Backs

8-10 reps

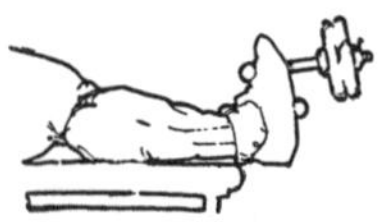

1 Set

Foot Inward Rocks

8-10 reps

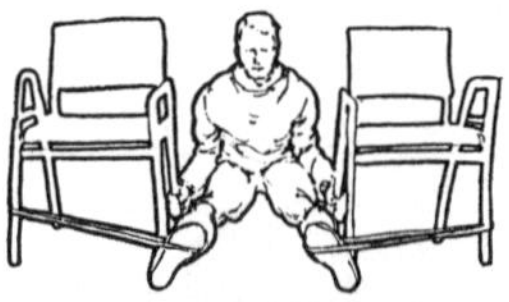

1 Set

Foot Outward Rocks

8-10 reps

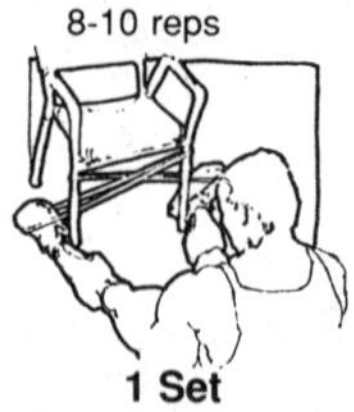

1 Set

LEVEL 1

Single Leg C.R.

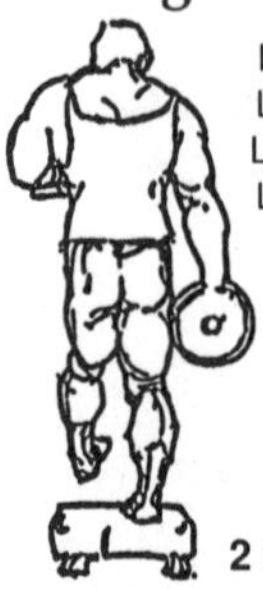

LS0: 6-8 reps
LSI: 4-6 reps
LBO: 6-8 reps
LBI: 4-6 reps

2 Sets

Donkey C.R.

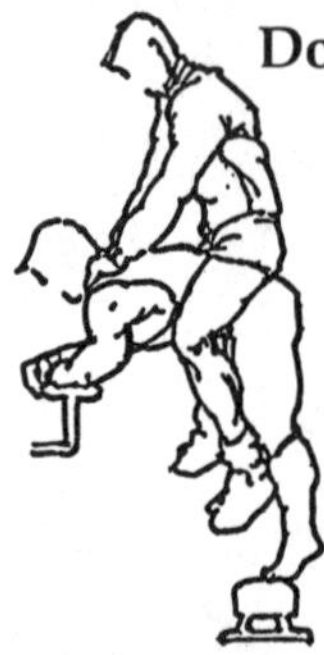

LS0: 6-8 reps
LSI: 4-6 reps
LBO: 6-8 reps
LBI: 4-6 reps

Calf Rock-ups

20 secs.

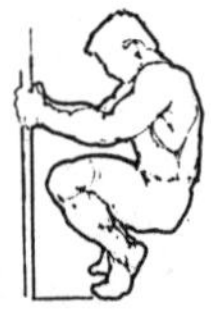

1 Compound Set

Seated Toe Pull-Backs

8-10 reps

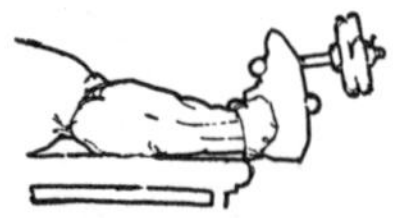

2 Sets

LEVEL 2

Single Leg C.R.

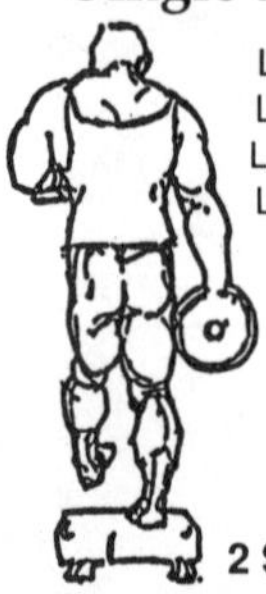

LS0: 6-8 reps
LSI: 4-6 reps
LBO: 6-8 reps
LBI: 4-6 reps

2 Sets

Donkey C.R.

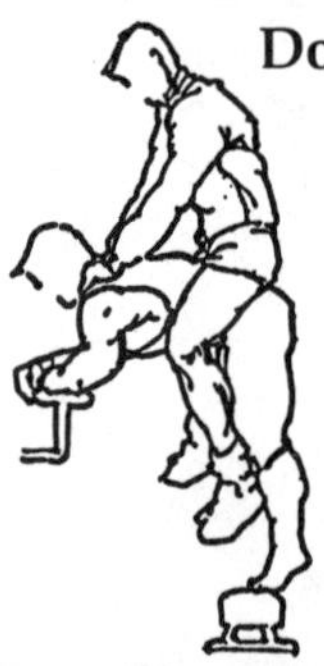

LS0: 6-8 reps
LSI: 4-6 reps
LBO: 6-8 reps
LBI: 4-6 reps

Calf Rock-ups

20 secs.

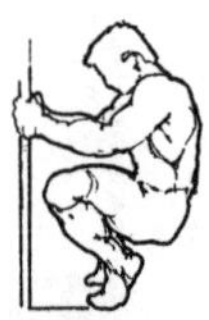

2 Compound Sets

Seated Toe Pull-Backs

8-10 reps

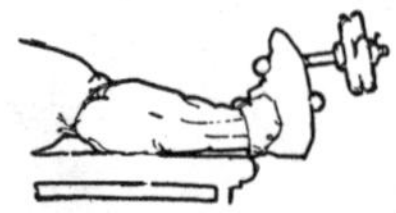

3 Sets

WARMUP

Standing Toe Pull-Backs

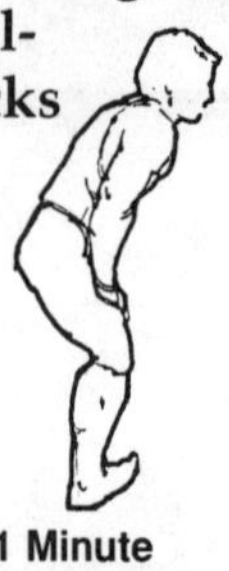

1 Minute

Calf Bounces

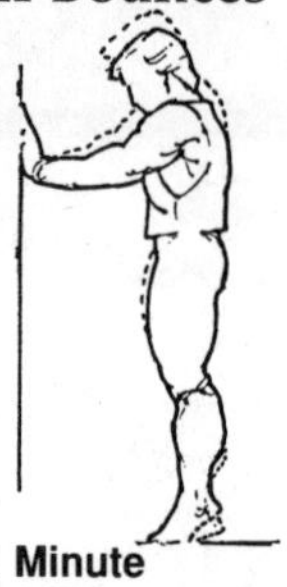

1 Minute

Footwork Speed/ Ankle Stability Routines *Illustrated*

Foot Inward Rocks

8-10 reps

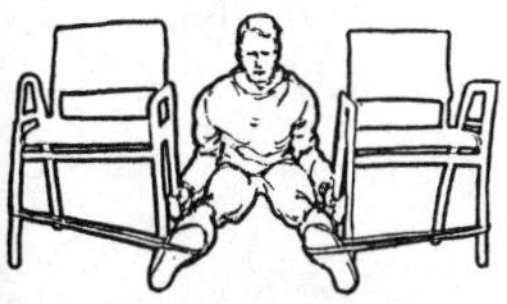

2 Sets

Foot Outward Rocks

8-10 reps

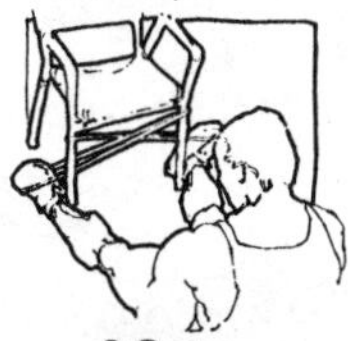

2 Sets

Foot Inward Rocks

8-10 reps

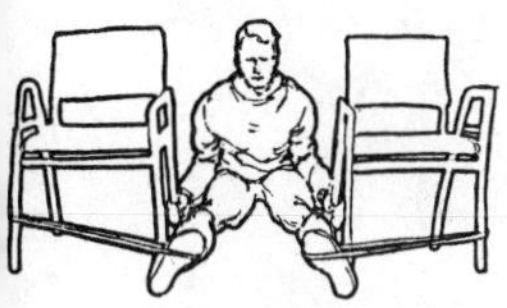

3 Sets

Foot Outward Rocks

8-10 reps

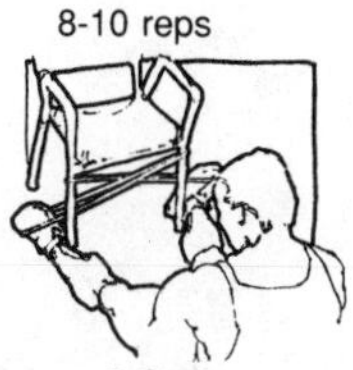

3 Sets

Begin all levels with the **Warmup** routine illustrated at the bottom of the previous page.

End all levels with the **Stretch** routine illustrated below.

STRETCH

Single Leg C.S.

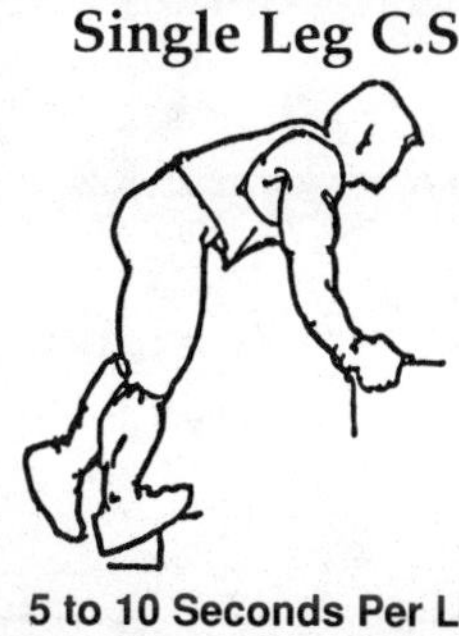

5 to 10 Seconds Per Leg

Toes Pointed C.S.

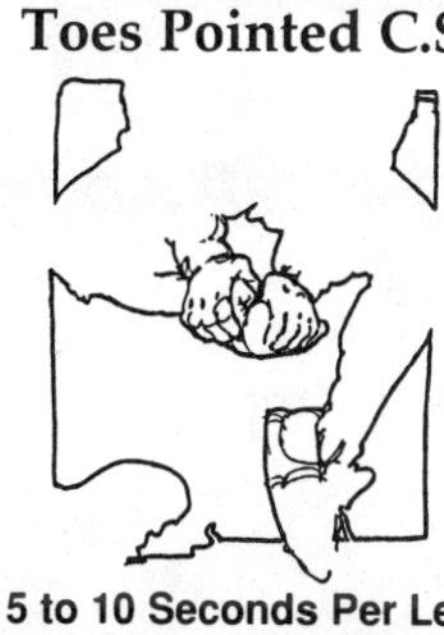

5 to 10 Seconds Per Leg

Ankle Rocked-In C.S.

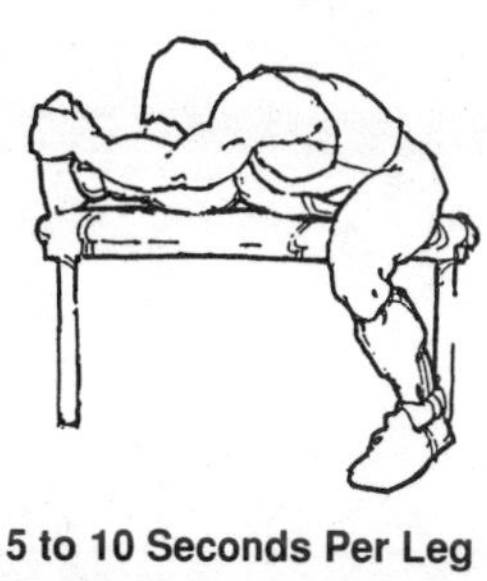

5 to 10 Seconds Per Leg

HOW MUCH, HOW OFTEN

Beginners should start with the Level A routine. Those who have been training calves for at least two months can start with Level 1. In either case, limit lower leg work to no more than three workouts per week; we recommend two. Reason: Muscle takes a full thirty-six hours to recover from a severe overload. Allowing less time than that between heavy training sessions for the same body part can actually lead to diminished results.

If possible, arrange your workout schedule to allow at least one day *after* **Maximum Calves** before working legs. Doing **Maximum Calves** the day *before*—or worse, immediately before—legs decreases calf stability enough to seriously increase your risk of knee and ankle injury. The best time to do **Maximum Calves** is immediately *after* legs. This allows maximum recovery time before the next leg workout.

Likewise, martial artists and other athletes who do the **Maximum Calves** routine before doing footwork-oriented training increase their risk of injury. Skill training should come first, followed by **Maximum Calves.**

(Note: Ditto running and jogging. Both rely heavily on leg stability, and so should be performed prior to the **Maximum Calves** routines. Furthermore, bear in mind the combined stresses of running plus leg work plus calf training can predispose you to overuse injuries such as shin splints. If your overall workout involves all three, watch for the nagging pains indicative of overuse. Back off if you experience them.)

Remember to abide by the guideline for the amount of weight to use: The proper amount will allow you move through the full range of motion for the muscle involved for all but the last one or two reps of each set. Those it will render nearly impossible.

Happy training!

EXAMPLES OF OPTIMUM SEQUENCING

If you work your whole body three days a week, do the **Maximum Calves** routines *after* the legs portion of your routine. If you don't do legs, do the **Maximum Calves** routines at the end of your workout.

MONDAY	WEDNESDAY	FRIDAY
Legs	Legs	Legs
Maximum Calves	**Maximum Calves**	**Maximum Calves**
Calf stretches	Calf stretches	Calf stretches

If you use a split routine (different body parts on different days), try to leave as much time between your calves and legs workouts as possible.

Six-day split — each body part 3 times per week

MONDAY	TUESDAY	WEDNESDAY	THURSDAY	FRIDAY	SATURDAY
Lower body **Maximum Calves** Calf stretches	Upper body	Lower body **Maximum Calves** Calf stretches	Upper body	Lower body **Maximum Calves** Calf stretches	Upper body

Six-day split — each body part 2 times per week

MONDAY	TUESDAY	WEDNESDAY	THURSDAY	FRIDAY	SATURDAY
Lower body **Maximum Calves** Calf stretches	Part of upper body	Rest of upper body	Lower body **Maximum Calves** Calf stretches	Part of upper body	Rest of upper body

Four-day split — each body part 2 times per week

MONDAY	TUESDAY	WEDNESDAY	THURSDAY	FRIDAY	SATURDAY
Lower body **Maximum Calves** Calf stretches	Upper body	rest	Lower body **Maximum Calves** Calf stretches	Upper body	rest

☆ ☆ ☆

GLOSSARY

Balanced Development: Proportional development of the strength of each of the muscles of an opposing muscle group pair at some joint (e.g. biceps/triceps).

Compound Set: Two exercises for the *same* muscle or muscle group performed back-to-back without rest. (Compare *Superset.*)

Dorsiflexion: Bending the ankle so the forefoot moves up toward the shin—the opposite of *plantar flexion*.

Fatigue/Tension Level: The degree of exhaustion of a muscle at any given point during exercise.

Fatigue/Tension Principle: A concept that interrelates fatigue and tension and the effect of varying these during exercise.

Fatigue/Tension Threshold: The minimum Fatigue/Tension level necessary for muscle growth.

Functional Strength: The ability of the body to bring a coordinated muscular effort to bear on external resistance in everyday situations, such as moving a refrigerator.

Functional Strength Exercise: Exercises that most closely duplicate movements in everyday life.

Giant Set: Three or more exercises for the same body part performed back-to-back without rest.

Interdependency of Muscle Groups: The principle stating that individual muscles never act alone.

Interdependency Principle: The principle stating that, if a muscle is going to be called upon to function as a helping muscle, or *synergist*, it should not be worked as prime mover prior to functioning as synergist.

Leverage: The mechanical advantage provided by position.

Load: The opposition to motion provided by weight.

Optimization: Maximizing output for a given input.

Overloading: Forcing a muscle to act against resistance greater than that which it can easily overcome.

Plantar Flexion: Bending the ankle so the forefoot moves down away from the shin—the opposite of *dorsiflexion.*

Pronation, ankle: A combination of ankle *eversion* (the bottom of the foot rolling outward) and *abduction* (the forefoot moving away from the body's centerline).

Resistance: The opposition to motion resulting from the combined effect of load and leverage.

Superset: Two exercises, one each for each of the muscle groups in an *opposing* pair (e.g. biceps/triceps), performed back-to-back without rest. (Compare *Compound Set.*)

Supination, ankle: A combination of ankle *inversion* (the bottom of the foot rolling inward) and *adduction* (the forefoot moving in toward the body's centerline).

Synergism: Combining elements to create a whole greater than just the sum of those elements.

Tension: Muscular contractile force.

Timing: (Also called *pace.*) The combination of rep speed, rests between sets, and rests between exercises.

☆ ☆ ☆

About our other courses:

Secrets of Advanced Bodybuilders

What **Legendary Abs** and **SynerAbs** do for abdominal conditioning, **Secrets of Advanced Bodybuilders** does for your whole workout! **Secrets** explains how to apply the Synergism principle to training back, chest, delts, biceps, triceps, quads, and hamstrings. It unlocks the secrets of the Optimum Workout, and shows you how to develop the best routines for *you*—with your particular goals, strengths, and body structure.

Get the *ultimate* program. Plus, learn... ❑ a new back exercise that will pile on the mass and increase power without putting harmful stress on your lower back ❑ a technique for making Leg Extensions 200% more intense by targeting both inner *and outer* quads ❑ the shift in position that cranks Pull-Up and Pull-Down exercises to 3 times normal intensity ❑ a *body weight* tricep exercise that will be "a growing experience" even for someone who's been training for years ❑ a *body weight* lat exercise that will mass up your back faster than you would have believed possible ❑ a special shoulder set that's more effective than most entire delt routines—also—❑ the best way to integrate your other athletic endeavors—running, cycling, stretching, mountain climbing, martial arts, etc.—into your routine to create the optimum overall program ❑ techniques for maximizing the effectiveness of *all* exercises you do, not just those in the course...and much, much more! *Stop working harder than you need to to get the results you want. Put the **Secrets of Advanced Bodybuilders** to work for you today! 158 pp. Over 300 illustrations.*

Secrets of Advanced Bodybuilders, Supplement #1

New breakthroughs in sports research are happening all the time. With the **Secrets** course as its foundation, the SUPPLEMENT series provides the most complete and up-to-date training resource available. Supplement #1 features a new 5-day split based on a unique three-week cycle that reduces workout time and minimizes the risk of overtraining. You'll also learn: ❑ optimum use of the jettison and pyramiding techniques (when these are effective, when not, how they fit into the **Secrets** routines) ❑ altering rep and set numbers to affect tendon or muscular strength, local muscular endurance, or speed ❑ machines vs. free weights and the best way to use both ❑ Exercise SetPoint, a brand-new concept integral to getting maximum results in minimum time. *All this, and a lot more! A 24 p. illustrated manual.*

Legendary Abs

The original. Featuring the Synergism principle, **Legendary Abs** guarantees rock-hard, well-defined Abs in just 6 minutes a day! See results within two weeks, or your money back. Not isometrics or some other supposed shortcut, **Legendary Abs** is just good science applied to bodybuilding. Over 80,000 copies sold worldwide! *A 24 p. illustrated manual.*

SynerAbs: 6 Minutes to a Flatter Stomach

Women's edition of the **Legendary Abs** program. Guarantees a firm, well-toned midsection in just 6 minutes a day! Ten levels of routines from beginning to advanced. *A 24 p. illustrated manual.*

Beyond Legendary Abs: A Synergistic Guide to *Legendary Abs* and *SynerAbs*

We know the serious bodybuilder is always reaching for greater gains. Letter after letter, our readers unanimously ask: "How can I go *further*?" The answer is in **Beyond Legendary Abs**—a new performance guide specially designed to supplement our phenomenally successful **Legendary Abs** and **SynerAbs** programs. It's the closest thing we can offer to a personal trainer! **Beyond** is not just for advanced bodybuilders! It's just as useful for the **beginner**, trying to get the most out of the program, or the **intermediate** on level 5, trying to break through a plateau. It's a detailed performance guide designed to maximize the efficiency of your training **at any level.** Now is the time to go *beyond! A 24 p. illustrated manual.*

SynerShape: A Scientific Weight Loss Guide

We're surrounded by weight loss myths. Crash diets. Spot reducing. Exotic herbs. Still, most plans fail, and most people who lose weight gain it back again. Is there really an honest, effective solution? **Yes!** **SynerShape** represents the next generation in awareness of how the body gains and metabolizes fat. It synthesizes the most recent findings on nutrition, exercise, and psychology into a TOTAL program, offering you the tools you need to shape the body you want. **SynerShape** works. Let it work for *you! A 24 p. illustrated manual.*

The Psychology of Weight Loss

This special program-on-tape picks up where **SynerShape** leaves off. Noted psychologist Carol Landesman explores eating problems and *solutions* based on the latest research into human behavior and metabolism. Then, through a series of exercises, she helps you begin to heal the emotional conflicts behind your weight problem. **The Psychology of Weight Loss** is a unique program that brings the power of the therapy process into the privacy of your home. *A 90-minute guided introspection. On audio cassette.*

SynerStretch: For Total Body Flexibility...FAST!

Two programs in one: Both deliver lower and upper body flexibility in less than 8 minutes a day! **SynerStretch A** is for you if you need to maintain your flexibility. Originally designed for martial artists—who depend on extreme flexibility— **SynerStretch A** will also help bodybuilders, dancers, and other athletes stay flexible in less than *5 minutes per workout.* A great way to end a training session of any kind! **SynerStretch B** is for you if you need to increase your flexibility. Not only does it take less than 8 minutes, but because it makes use of a new, relatively unknown technique (Isometric Agonist Contraction/Relaxation), it eliminates most of the pain usually associated with stretching. It works! When you order **SynerStretch**, you get both programs in one manual for just $9.95. Get loose, and stay loose with **SynerStretch**. *A 28 p. illustrated manual.*

Power ForeArms!

Here at last is a program that specifically targets the hard-to-develop forearm muscles. Like all Health For Life programs, **Power ForeArms!** is based on the Synergism principle, and yields maximum results in minimum time. Designed for serious bodybuilders and martial artists, **Power ForeArms!** will help you build strong, solid, massive forearms in just 7 to 12 minutes, twice a week. Give **Power ForeArms!** a try. *A 32 p. illustrated manual.*

For price and order information, call **1-800-874-5339**
(in California, call **1-800-523-9983**), or write us at...

Health For Life
Suite 483
8033 Sunset Blvd.
Los Angeles, CA 90046